Healing Trauma with Yoga

Go From Surviving to Thriving with Mind-Body Techniques

Beth Shaw

BLUE
RIVER
PRESS

INDIANAPOLIS, INDIANA

Healing Trauma with Yoga:
Go From Surviving to Thriving with Mind-Body Techniques
Copyright © Beth Shaw, 2019

Published by Blue River Press
Indianapolis, Indiana
www.brpressbooks.com

Distributed by Cardinal Publishers Group
A Tom Doherty Company, Inc.
www.cardinalpub.com

ISBN: 978-1-68157-777-7

Cover Design And Book Design: Rick Korab, Korab Company Design
Editors: Danielle Bernabe and Dani McCormick
Photographs: Luciana Pampalone

Printed in the United States of America

10 9 8 7 6 5 4 3 2 1   19 20 21 22 23 24 25 26 27 28

We all breathe the same

universal life-force energy.

May we find healing together,

in unity and community,

As one.

Namaste

TABLE OF CONTENTS

*"Yoga teaches us to cure what need not be
endured and endure what cannot be cured."*

—B. K. S. Iyengar

To be human is to have suffered countless times throughout a life journey.
When the pain strikes so deeply that it overwhelms the ability to cope, it
transforms into trauma. What is trauma? The Greeks defined *trávma* or
τραύμα as a 'wound,' indeed one that can pierce to the core an individual's
mind, body and spirit, often impairing the ability to feel joy and to function
optimally.

Trauma itself is in the eyes of the beholder. The same life event can be
perceived very differently from one person to another when viewed through
the lens of that individual's life experience. Genetics and environment play
major roles in shaping reactions to the full spectrum of life challenges, which
can include any form of abuse as well as grief and loss, difficult relationships,
distressing world events, and health conditions. Clearly, severe physical
and mental abuse can be profoundly traumatic for most people, burdening
them with fear, distrust, difficulty connecting with others, and constant,
exhausting hypervigilance.

At the heart of optimal trauma management is the ability to practice
stress-resilience. This means that, when an individual perceives a stress that
is deeply wounding, instead of defaulting to potentially self-destructive
trauma behavior, she finds a way to navigate the challenge by productively
adapting and adjusting to her circumstances. Thus, the key to survival in the
face of traumatic experiences is the daily practice of stress-resilience through
regrouping, re-centering, resetting, and rejuvenating.

What better way to become mentally, physically, and spiritually strong
than through the regular practice of yoga?

No one is immune to life's stresses and traumas. Some are fortunate
and are stress-resilient enough to adapt and adjust to mental and physical
wounds inflicted during the course of their lives. Others become entangled in

trauma's aftermath, struggling to survive under the dark clouds of anguish and distress. In the end, we all live in recovery, as we confront each day's tasks and challenges. Yoga, then, can become a key part of our ongoing healing and recovery process, a life-course that continues until our final breath.

Central to experiencing yoga is the celebration of profoundly self-compassionate holistic connections between mind and body. This counters one of the principal consequences of trauma—mental and physical dissociation, a common coping mechanism to numb incessant pain and angst. The gentle yet powerful yoga *asanas* can help heal trauma-related disconnects. Simply learning the *pranayama* breath practices can be a miraculous event as one feels the body accepting each breath through the expanding chest and abdomen, all the while awakening to the mindful gratitude of just being. To address the need for more trauma focus, the yoga community has begun to develop new training and educational platforms to include trauma-sensitive and trauma-based yoga practices.

Recently, scientists have begun to study the relationship between yoga practice and post-traumatic stress disorder (PTSD) in a variety of populations. One study of military veterans noted:

> "There was significant improvement in PTSD hyperarousal symptoms and overall sleep quality as well as daytime dysfunction related to sleep.... These results suggest that this yoga program may be an effective adjunctive therapy for improving hyperarousal symptoms of PTSD including sleep quality. This study demonstrates that the yoga program is acceptable [and] feasible, and that there is good adherence in a Veteran population."

Renowned trauma therapist Dr. Bessel Van Der Kolk, Director of the Trauma Research Foundation, was one of the first scientists to utilize yoga in both trauma therapy recovery, as well as research studies. In studying the neuroscience of self-awareness in women with chronic PTSD, Van der Kolk found that a twenty-week extended yoga treatment resulted in significant reductions in the symptoms of PTSD and mind-body dissociation. In his seminal text *The Body Keeps the Score: Brain, Mind and Body in the Healing of Trauma*, Van der Kolk notes:

Traumatized people chronically feel unsafe inside their bodies: The past is alive in the form of gnawing interior discomfort. Their bodies are constantly bombarded by visceral warning signs, and, in an attempt to control these processes, they often become expert at ignoring their gut feelings and in numbing awareness of what is played out inside. They learn to hide from their selves.

Individuals afflicted with PTSD frequently do not feel safe in their bodies. They are easily triggered by any form of sensory stimulation, especially touch. When this occurs, immediate panic and anxiety ensue. Trauma-informed yoga instructors are keenly aware of this critical threat to the wellbeing of their yoga student. Now students can take that power into their own hands.

Beth Shaw's book *Healing Trauma with Yoga* is an essential read for anyone who has experienced trauma, practices yoga, or teaches yoga.

This book is very timely. Today, individuals are becoming more aware of the effect of long-term stress and trauma on their mind-body. I'm certain that women and men who live with PTSD will be greatly relieved to know that there is a safe haven, a yoga class led by a well-trained, compassionate, understanding instructor who is sensitive to the presence of their ongoing and often tenuous healing process. YogaFit has trainings specifically geared toward trauma so instructors are well-equipped and compassionate. This book gives the tools to help people heal themselves. In this book, beyond just tools and techniques, Beth shares insights into the world of trauma, including her own personal story. She genuinely understands the desperate need for traumatized people to develop trust with their yoga instructors and themselves and their own practice. It is from this profound passion and desire to be of service to people who are seeking help from their life traumas that Beth Shaw has gifted all of us with a blueprint for recovery and healing through yoga and mind-body tools.

Pamela Peeke

MD, MPH, FACP, FACSM

Assistant Professor of Medicine, University of Maryland

New York Times bestselling author of *Body for Life for Women*

*"Yoga is the journey of the self,
through the self, to the self."*
—Bhagavad Gita

While collecting stories of trauma and healing for this book, I was moved to tears on numerous occasions by not only the amount of submissions but the variety of ways in which trauma occurs. I realized both the importance of sharing my own story and the courage it takes anyone to do the same. Although limited to a certain allotment of pages, much like the journey of healing, these pages could be endless. Trauma varies from person to person. The path to healing is fortunately a very wide one with many options. My own journey to heal trauma has been ongoing for more than forty years and is still in process.

At age three, my parents moved us from New York City, where I was born, to live on a boat. My father, a World War II veteran who was seventeen years the senior of my mother (his fourth wife), had a dream to retire early and tour Europe by the sea. We spent the next three years cruising the canals of France, Italy, and the Mediterranean Sea until the money ran out and we had to return to the United States. It was during *savasana* (final resting pose) eighteen years later that I had my first and only memory of my father sexually molesting me on that very boat while my mother was out shopping. Looking back now, everything makes sense: the migraines and headaches I developed at age six; the nightly stomach pains at age seven; the alcohol use in my late teens that continued sporadically longer than I care to admit; the history of relationships with people with addiction; the lack of self-esteem despite my external successes; and my own personal struggles with depression and emotional dysregulation.

My father received a purple heart after being shot in the leg in Italy during the war, my bedtime stories were all his war stories. I now realize that his love of martinis, which he started drinking daily in the midafternoon, were his way of medicating himself from trauma and Post Traumatic Stress Disorder

(PTSD). My father's unhealthy lifestyle, which included smoking two packs of cigarettes per day, led him to an early death at age seventy-three.

My mother was the first-generation daughter of Hungarian immigrants. Her father was a rageaoholic who beat her and her brother with a belt every Saturday night. He was a dictatorial narcissistic personality who ran the home with a heavy hand—from counting the spoons to becoming irate over the vegetable to meat ratio served at dinner. My mother inherited these traits, which resulted in a lot of reactions and fighting in our household. As a result of this childhood, my mother exhibited a lack of empathy, attachment, and compassion. She probably had Borderline Personality Disorder but was undiagnosed. I was constantly in fear of her anger, never knowing when she would erupt next, or what would set her off. The littlest things would enrage her. I also suffered from her consistent invalidation of my feelings. Now that being said, I have to express my gratitude for the example she set for me as a hard-working business woman, a phenomenal cook, and for providing me with the opportunity to start on my path of fitness when she joined the YMCA when my parents divorced. After that point I was pretty much left to raise myself in New York City at thirteen.

Self-care was not new to me. I taught myself guided meditation at age six to rid myself of those blinding migraine headaches as no one in my household seemed to want to help. As an only child, I learned coping skills early on. Picturing myself on a beach or the forest combined with breathing techniques seemed to clear the headaches up, even though I would sometimes vomit before that happened. The migraines would start with bright white lights shooting across my eyes and progress rapidly from there. Self-taught guided meditation was my one and only way out of pain.

Fortunately, I also discovered the gym at age fifteen, and exercise quickly became a tool for stress management.

Although I've been practicing yoga poses since childhood, my own formal practice did not start until I moved to Los Angeles right after college. My first teacher had also healed herself with yoga. Rene Taylor, who was ninety-three when I met her, had cancer in the late 1960s. She moved to Rishikesh, India where, ironically, my school YogaFit now brings people every year.

Rishikesh is the birthplace of yoga, which originated in the Ganges River Basin over 6,000 years ago. Rene cured herself with yoga, meditation, vegetarian diet, and Ayurvedic medicine (the oldest medicine system in the world). Rene then came back to the United States and began writing books on yoga. I feel like in some way, Rene transferred Shaktipat (a spiritual energy that is passed from one person to another) to me during those early years of my practice. Following in her lineage four books and twenty-two years of educating and bringing people to yoga later, YogaFit has touched the lives of millions on this planet.

The path of yoga has been a very winding one for me personally, instigated in this lifetime by the need to heal myself. Yoga has been a gateway for me, opening me up to the possibility of healing and discovery in many different ways. Yoga has literally saved my life on many occasions. It is what I've returned to with vigor during some of the most difficult times and what I have come to rely on for a day-to-day practice. Yoga incorporates so much more than just physical poses. Yoga is a mindset and a lifestyle.

The Essence of YogaFit resonates with me today more than it did over twenty-two years ago when I sat down to write the first YogaFit manual. That essence is simply:

- Breathing
- Feeling
- Listening to our bodies
- Letting go of judgement, expectation, and competition
- Staying present in the moment.

Throughout this book, we will learn how to apply these principles to ourselves while dealing with PTSD, trauma, addiction, anxiety, and depression. We will use the essence as our mantra to stay open, curious, positive, and present to our unique and individual process of healing.

I am grateful to the practice of yoga; it has directed my life and kept me on a steady path of growth, transformation, and evolution. I will readily admit that during the times in my life where I abandoned my yoga practice, bad things happened and poor choices led to some additional adult trauma. Fortunately, those opportunities have allowed me to course-correct, find a deeper place in my practice, and learn more about healing by using myself as the test case. I will only advocate for something I have tried and found positive results from.

Therapists, twelve-step groups, plant medicine, shamans, astrologers, energy healers, body workers, psychiatrists, medication, supplements, John of God, soul readers—I've done a lot of experimenting. I can honestly say that taking the power into your own hands for your healing is your most empowered course, *always*. Yoga gives you that power.

I am now in a place where I know I will stay for my remaining years on this planet—focused, content, healthy, committed to my life's work, and leading a purpose-driven life.

The yogic path offers so many options and solutions. My hope is that this book provides you with insight into trauma, tools for healing, and a broad roadmap for you to live your best life from today forward.

May you heal yourself and heal others.
Namaste,
Beth

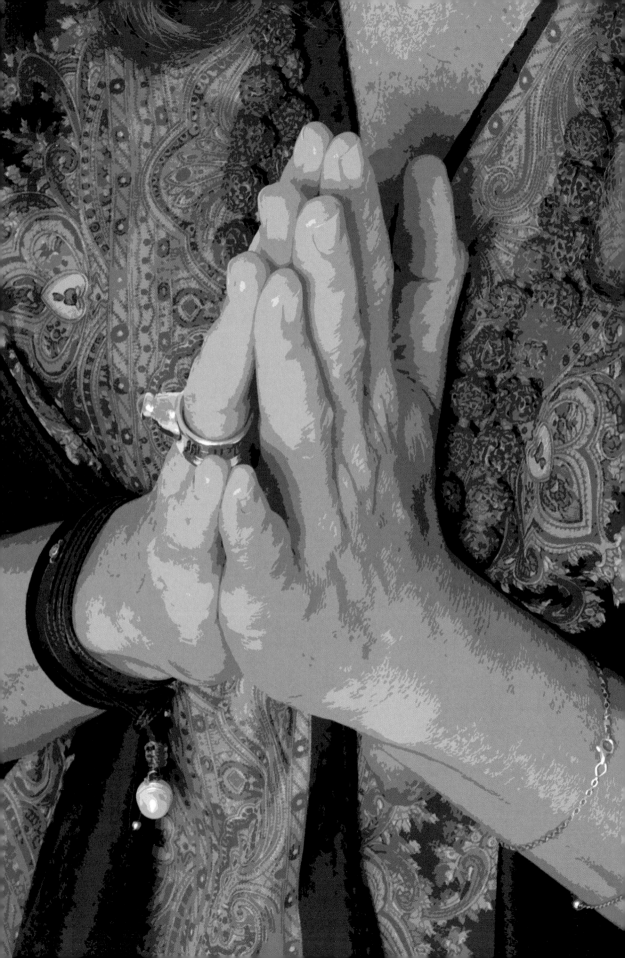

CHAPTER 1

Trauma Today

"I am the fresh taste of water, the light of the sun and moon; I am the sacred syllable OM, the sound in ether, and the ability in man."

—Bhagavad Gita 7:8

What Is Trauma and What Does It Look Like?

Having a better understanding of trauma and the impact that a traumatic event makes to the brain and body can give insight into the healing process. When a traumatic event occurs, your life is altered through the physical and mental changes that happen during and after your experience. In order to heal trauma, we must learn to identify our patterns of thought and behavior, especially when those patterns are new to you. It is important to be open to the idea that there are unresolved "issues in your tissues" that are creating the post-traumatic injuries, illness, or events in our lives. Knowing why these changes occur, and how your life and well-being are altered drastically by trauma, can bring meaning to the recovery process and help your body and brain recalibrate once again.

The ACE Test

The ACE Test, Adverse Childhood Experiences Test and Health Outcomes, is a wonderful self-assessment test to determine where you fall on the trauma scale. Pause right now before you go any further in this book and answer these ten questions. I wish that this test was in existence and that I had the opportunity to take it as I neared adulthood. This is something I believe everyone should have access to and take at least by the time they reach adulthood because if people knew about this, it could shed light on their journey. Feel free to share it with you clients, family and friends.

While you were growing up, during your first eighteen years of life:

1. Did a parent or other adult in the household often swear at you, insult you, put you down, or humiliate you or act in a way that made you afraid that you might be physically hurt?
   Yes   No

2. Did a parent or other adult in the household often push, grab, slap, or throw something at you or ever hit you so hard that you had marks or were injured?
   Yes   No

3. Did an adult or person at least five years older than you ever touch or fondle you or have you touch their body in a sexual way or try to or actually have oral, anal, or vaginal sex with you?
   Yes   No

4. Did you often feel that no one in your family loved you or thought you were important or special or your family didn't look out for each other, feel close to each other, or support each other?
   Yes   No

5. Did you often feel that you didn't have enough to eat, had to wear dirty clothes, and had no one to protect you or your parents were too drunk or high to take care of you or take you to the doctor if you needed it?
   Yes   No

6. Were your parents ever separated or divorced?
   Yes   No

7. Was your mother or stepmother often pushed, grabbed, slapped, or had something thrown at her or sometimes or often kicked, bitten, hit with a fist, or hit with something hard or ever repeatedly hit over at least a few minutes or threatened with a gun or knife?
   Yes   No

8. Did you live with anyone who was a problem drinker or alcoholic or who used street drugs?
   Yes   No

9. Was a household member depressed or mentally ill or did a household member attempt suicide?

   Yes   No

10. Did a household member go to prison?

   Yes   No

Now, count all your yeses and take a look at the following. In comparison to those reporting a zero on their ACE score, individuals with four or more on their ACE score had significantly greater odds of reporting the following:

- Ischemic Heart Disease   2.2 percent
- Any Cancer   1.9 percent
- Chronic bronchitis or emphysema   3.9 percent
- Stroke   2.4 percent
- Diabetes   1.6 percent
- Ever Attempting Suicide   12.2 percent
- Severe Obesity   1.6 percent
- Two or more weeks of depressed mood in past year   4.6 percent
- Ever using illicit drug   4.7 percent
- Ever injecting drug   10.3 percent
- Current smoking   2.2 percent
- Ever having sexually transmitted disease   2.5 percent

Typical Causes of Trauma

There are many things that can lead to trauma, and each experience is unique to the individual, along with the side effects that accompany it. Trauma can be a direct emotional or physical experience, from childhood or adulthood, a onetime event, or ongoing exposure.

Transgenerational trauma, which is trauma passed down from first generation survivors to offspring generations through PTSD behaviors, is also common. Often times this occurs when the behaviors of the survivor are observed by the children. They sense the stress, absorb it, and then adjust with the symptoms. Living in a household surrounded by constant PTSD symptoms can become a great burden to those who were not directly impacted by a traumatic event. Furthermore, when a survivor lives with symptoms, their behavior may change, which could potentially include anger or rage. For instance, the trauma cycle often continues in the survivor if the survivor doesn't move on to heal from the symptoms..A child who experienced sexual abuse, may grow up with behavioral issues that evolve into projected actions, such as abuse onto someone else.

With the world becoming "smaller" through TV and the internet, we can even experience vicarious trauma as ever-rising numbers of traumatic and violent events are brought into our living room and seen over and over again. Daily exposure to images of violence, natural disasters, kidnappings, terrorist attacks, and even horror movies are creating a culture of trauma.

Some typical sources of trauma are:
- War experience
- Sexual abuse
- Emotional and physical abuse
- Mass shootings
- Medical trauma
- Traumatic loss (accident, murder, etc.)
- Vicarious trauma
- Natural disasters
- Childhood neglect
- Environmental endangerment

In some cases, trauma can be caused by seemingly innocuous events such as:
- Illness or major disease, such as cancer
- Medical or dental procedures
- Minor fender benders
- Falls or minor injuries
- Sudden loud noises (especially in children and babies)
- Birth stress for mom or baby
- Prolonged immobilization, such as after an injury
- Exposure to extreme temperatures
- Any stressful or overwhelming experience

Impact of Trauma

People living with residual trauma are continually getting ready for attack or life-altering event. I find myself hypervigilant more times than I would like, and when someone is preoccupied by a real or imagined threat, the resulting fear, rage, or disappointment will be reflected in the body. Research shows that trauma survivors suffer more illness, as referenced in *Overcoming Trauma Through Yoga* by Emerson, et al. Muscle tension, disease, and injury are physical manifestations of this preoccupation.

Why, though, does trauma have such a severe impact? Because of the way it affects, and ultimately, rewires the brain. When the brain goes into stress or is stuck in stress, it leads to physical changes and a complicated ripple of life-altering symptoms.

In the animal world, animals "shake off" the freeze response caused by a life threat. When animals suffer trauma, it has been documented that they will literally shake it off, which helps the animal discharge the energy of the traumatic event. I watch my dog Bentley, a rescue who has puppyhood trauma, do this often as he gets triggered by brightly-lit neon signs, overhead scaffolding, awnings, and hats and sunglasses on men with uniforms. He shakes it off, and I encourage it by saying, "Shake it off, Boo. Shake it off."

The term "shaking like a leaf" is commonly used to describe a reaction to a frightening situation. Shaking or trembling, which comes from the limbic brain (the part of the brain that holds emotions), sends a signal that the danger has passed and that the fight-or-flight system can turn off. The action is literally finishing the nervous system response to release the traumatic experience from the body. Animals often die if they are unable to shake off the trauma, but in humans it may evolve into mental or physical illness.

Humans also shake off trauma, but the problem comes when something prevents the nervous system from completing its natural, survival-based response, such as being held down, held against your will, or being immobilized (duty requirement in military or via medication from an unwitting medical attendant), for example. In these cases, the experience can become stored in the body, resulting in mental or physical illness—or both—and can lead to a diagnosis of Post-Traumatic Stress Disorder (PTSD).

Impact of Trauma to the Brain

After a traumatic event, one that represents a threat to personal safety, the brain and body are transformed. The threat evokes a physical and emotional reaction in the person experiencing the event, which activates our Sympathetic Nervous System (SNS)—also known as fight or flight, a necessary and important survival response. After trauma, the SNS remains activated, keeping the body and mind in high alert. The brain and nervous system become stuck in trauma and are rewired in a way that makes healing a challenge. According to neuroscientist Paul D. MacLean, the brain is made up of three parts, known as the Triune Brain Model:

1. Reptilian (brain stem): responsible for survival instincts and autonomic body processes.
2. Mammalian (limbic, midbrain): processes emotions and conveys sensory relays.
3. Neomammalian (cortex, forebrain): controls cognitive processing, decision-making, learning, memory, and inhibitory functions.

The reptilian brain is activated during trauma and alerts the body to react and go into survival mode. This is when the SNS prepares for fight or flight. In a non-threatening situation, the brain and body are able to alleviate this reaction and shift back to its normal functioning—also known as "top-down" control of how our brains make use of information that has already been brought into the brain by one or more of the sensory systems. Top-down processing is a cognitive process that initiates with our thoughts, which then flow down to lower-level functions, such as the senses. Perception is driven by cognition. Your brain applies what it knows and what it expects to perceive, then fills in the blanks.

With trauma, however, the stress and hormones activated in the brain are stuck in survival mode and do not restore. The reptilian brain remains primed for threat and keeps the survivor in a reactive state, ultimately affecting other brain structures to react accordingly. When your brain is in constant stress mode, it trickles down and is normalized into the physical body, thus normalizing the tense behavior. And if the brain does not reset, some survivors develop PTSD.

There are biological and chemical changes that occur in the brain, which can literally shift your life, well-being, and reality as you know it. This is the post-traumatic brain. Symptoms, including intrusion, dissociation, numbness, and arousal (which we will dive deeper into in a bit) are then exhibited. It is jolting when all of a sudden your life has been impacted by trauma. It may feel like your reality and the person you once were are not the same after trauma. Survivors of trauma often feel out of control of their self, their mind, and their body. This can lead to an onslaught of challenges and symptoms that may be utterly overwhelming to handle on one's own or without the proper tools to help. When the brain dysregulates, the following chemical imbalances happen:

- Overstimulated amygdala: An almond-shaped mass located deep in the brain, the amygdala is responsible for survival-related threat identification and tagging memories with emotion. After trauma, the amygdala can get caught up in a highly alert and activated loop, during which it looks for and perceives threat everywhere.

- Underactive hippocampus: An increase in the stress hormone glucocorticoid kills cells in the hippocampus, which renders it less effective in making the synaptic connections necessary for memory consolidation. This interruption keeps both the body and mind stimulated in reactive mode as neither element receives the message that the threat has transformed into the past tense.

- Ineffective variability: The constant elevation of stress hormones interferes with the body's ability to regulate itself. The sympathetic nervous system remains highly activated leading to fatigue of the body and many of its systems, most notably the adrenal system.

Peptides and the Hypothalamus

When the brain deals with trauma in this matter, sometimes intense symptoms will develop.

Peptides are regular doses of a particular chemical release, an amino acid chain created by the hypothalamus. There is a peptide for every emotion manufactured by the hypothalamus and received by our cells. When we perceive an event in any way, the wires in our brain fire the signal to the hypothalamus to manufacture and release the chemical into our bloodstream. You may have heard the term "neurons that fire together, wire together."

Those who have suffered trauma are particularly susceptible to interpreting certain events as more trauma. The greater the emotional reaction to anything, the larger the dose of peptides that get made, released and distributed. Because the peptides are released into the cells, we feel them somatically. There are positive peptides and negative ones. When we relive a negative event in our mind, we release more negative peptides, and we can in fact become addicted to this peptide and then seek out situations that help these negative peptides to be released. When we don't rid our internal trauma, we get more of the same. Peptides are as addictive as any drug, and rats injected with peptides forgo food and self-care—just like a drug or alcohol addiction.

Even if we are doing a lot of self-work, if we allow ourselves to think about and relive the trauma, the brain fires off the electrical signal and the hypothalamus manufactures the peptide again and the downward spiral continues. We get more of the same.

Good peptides actually increase our cells ability to absorb nutrients and oxygen and help us look and feel great.

I continue retraining my brain by catching negative thoughts before they consume me (and my negative peptides), eating healthy foods, using advanced technology like the red light panels, my headstand machine, TrueDark glasses, magic weighted blankets, meditation, brain supplements, and living a joyous life with laugher, friends, music and dancing. See Additional Materials for coupon codes.

I believe it is imperative to understand our brains, peptides, addiction to them, the problem with negative thoughts and reliving trauma. We can be free, we only need to set ourselves free. Yes, it's a lot of work and it may seem overwhelming, but it is certainly worth it.

Evolution of Trauma, Its Diagnosis, and Treatment

In order to understand today's treatment used for trauma and post-traumatic stress disorder (PTSD), it is helpful and interesting to understand a little bit of its history. To witness how its treatment has evolved from shaming to compassion is a journey that has a fitting conclusion with the inclusion of yoga. Valuable windows into the evolution of PTSD treatment are soldiers and disaster victims. Clearly, war and disasters are not the only causes of trauma, but they are the most heavily-researched and funded. Symptoms of trauma are varied and diverse, but much of the treatment is similar.

It wasn't until the mid-1800s that physical and mental symptoms were linked with traumatic events. Mood disorders and other symptoms were sometimes labeled "hysteria" with "mysterious" origins. In the late 1800s, Jean-Martin Charcot, the father of modern neurology, identified a connection between common patterns of hysteria to traumatic stimulus. Freud, a student of Charcot's, later termed the phrase "traumatic neurosis;" he then formed a treatment of verbal expression combined with emotional discharge, believing that responses to trauma could be differentiated from the symptoms. In the early 1900s, Pierre Janet first described how a traumatic event and the intense emotional responses led to dissociation. Dissociation, where the mind and body connection can be broken, is a way that a trauma victim can step out of the experience to "survive."

According to the home page of the US Department of Veterans Affairs (VA), "Exposure a traumatic experience has always been a part of the human condition." Research and treatment for that trauma, though, really began around 1915 during World War I.

After World War I, trauma came more into focus when soldiers began describing symptoms such as tremors, tics, and gait problems, along with auditory and visual difficulties that seemed unexplainable. The term "flight into illness" was used to describe a theory of an internal conflict between fear and duty. The soldiers were described as having "conversion hysteria," and a number of terms were coined: "shell shocked," "war shock," "war psychoneurosis," and more. WWII brought more terms, including "battle fatigue" and "combat exhaustion." Soldiers who had seen and survived horrific events during war, as well as Holocaust survivors and prisoners of war, exhibited trauma-related symptoms.

Because the devastating effects of war presented themselves in such magnitude and with so many undiagnosed conditions, the governments of many countries, like Britain and the US, invested in research and treatment for the soldiers. Symptoms of PTSD definitely predated WWI, as did treatments and names. From shell shock to PTSD, trauma treatments have evolved from shock therapy to holistic approaches such as yoga and are recorded through the research and treatment of our veterans.

Treatment of trauma continued to evolve in the psychiatric field. In 1942, Wilfred Bion and John Rickman, psychiatrists in the army, developed what would later be called group therapy. Their goal was to create a leaderless group for soldier patients to talk in a safe space. This spawned a generation of group therapists for post-war "talk therapy."

In the 1950s, there emerged a new generation of psychiatric drugs to help combat the symptoms of PTSD, and the first approaches to cognitive behavioral therapy (CBT)—also known as cognitive therapy (CT)—thought that negative thoughts create negative emotions and actions that create additional pain to the sufferer of trauma. CBT looks to train the traumatized victim's brain to identify their fundamental negative thought patterns.

Albert Elis developed the early foundations of CBT called Rational Emotional Behavior Therapy (REBT). Elis proposed that each individual has a set of irrational assumptions about themselves and REBT is a therapy that encourages the patient to look at him or herself to examine their fears. Elis believed common irrational assumptions were the ideas that:

- One should be thoroughly competent at everything.
- It is catastrophic when things are not the way you want them to be.
- People have no control over their happiness.
- You need someone stronger than yourself to be dependent on.
- Your past history greatly influences your present life.

The American Psychiatric Association (APA) developed its first diagnostic manual, the *Diagnostic and Statistical Manual of Mental Disorders* (DSM) just after World War II, and the term "gross stress reaction" was used to describe the acute physiological responses following exposure to an extreme stressor. There was no mention of longer-lasting symptoms in that first DSM, nor the second edition published in 1968. It wasn't until after the Vietnam War that PTSD was included in the DSM-III. The next few additions of the DSM saw an ever-expanding definition of trauma and PTSD.

The latest information can be found in the DSM-V, which contains the most up-to-date criteria for diagnosing mental disorders, along with descriptive text providing a common language for clinicians to communicate about their patients.

It is clear in the many books on the topic of trauma and PTSD that experts believe that the diagnostic criteria do not begin to describe all of the possible scenarios for someone to experience trauma. Dr. Robert Scaer, in his book *The Body Bears the Burden: Trauma, Dissociation, and Disease*, which debuted in 2001, points out that many of the studies that give us the statistics and prevalence in our world today on trauma and PTSD only give us the tip of the iceberg. Trauma does not have to come from a single catastrophic event. What is traumatic and harmful to one person may be stimulating and exciting to another. Perception of threat, which is the root of trauma (your body going into fight or flight and getting stuck) is unique to each individual, past history, and circumstance. If we define traumatic stress by the response elicited, then we can say "any stressor sufficient enough to produce traumatic symptoms of re-experiencing, arousal, and avoidance should qualify as a traumatic event."

Last Few Decades

The last few decades have seen a number of traumatic events from 9/11 to wars and natural disasters affecting thousands of people to mass shootings and other violent crimes, including the Boston Marathon bombings. With these events now televised and reported 24/7, many people are transported right to the scene and thus are witness to trauma and at risk for trauma-related disorders such as PTSD. When we think about PTSD and trauma, we tend to think of experiencing firsthand major catastrophes involving life-or-death scenarios or events so horrific that those affected suffer various kinds of mental disturbances such as nightmares, sleep disturbances, anxiety, depression, and other symptoms. Trauma and PTSD are probably much more widespread due to the television and internet access that brings these events into our living rooms to be seen sometimes hundreds of times per day. During the Boston coverage, one morning show showed the bombing twenty-seven times in the first five minutes.

Traumatic stress and the resulting symptoms and diseases may be far more reaching in our world than many have realized. There are many types of trauma, some perhaps repressed in our memories from childhood and some resulting from seemingly "normal-life" events. We may suffer various symptoms or even recurring diseases or accidents that are perhaps evidence of unresolved trauma. Trauma can impact us in ways that may not show up for years. The statistics below are just those that meet the diagnostic criteria. Consider that there may be countless undiagnosed and borderline cases having effects on the health of our nation.

Below are some of the trauma and PTSD statistics, which I believe are vastly underreported:

- 7.7 million Americans over the age of eighteen suffer from PTSD.
- In one survey, 70 percent of people experienced a traumatic event.
- A study of adult women found 35.6 percent had experienced a crime, 14.3 percent a molestation or sexual assault, 13.4 percent a death of close relative or friend by murder, 12.7 percent a rape, and 10.3 percent a physical assault.[1]
- Three million children (one in twenty-five) experience some form of endangerment each year. One third of these are directly sexual, physical, or emotional.[2]
- One in four persons has been sexually assaulted in childhood according to Peter Levine, PhD, in *Healing Trauma*. Levine further goes on to say this is a conservative estimate.
- One in four have been directly affected by violence (interpersonal or community) by the time they are eighteen.[3]
- 1.3 million women and 835,000 men are physically assaulted by an intimate partner each year.
- Domestic violence is the leading cause of injury for women ages fifteen to forty-four (more than auto accidents, mugging, and cancer deaths combined).
- Suicide rate is increasing among the active duty Army, National Guard, and Reserve.[4] Preliminary data from the VA shows that the suicide rate for eighteen to twenty-nine-year-old male veterans who have left the military rose 26 percent from 2005 to 2007, and the rate climbed to record highs by 2012.

---

1 Resnick et al; *Journal of Consulting and Clinical Psychiatry,* 1993; 61:984-991
2 Emerson et al; *Overcoming Trauma Through Yoga*
3 Emerson et al; *Overcoming Trauma Through Yoga*
4 Department of Defense 2001

Post-traumatic Symptoms

While a lot of people are able to recover, a small but significant number go on to progress with serious complications. PTSD is a severe anxiety disorder that is usually diagnosed when symptoms last longer than one month and include re-experiencing trauma through flashbacks or nightmares, avoidance of stimuli associated with the trauma, increased arousal resulting in difficulty falling asleep, anger and hyper-vigilance, addiction, rage, and other effects. Complex PTSD is a more profound result of living in a world of neglect and maltreatment for a long period of time and the resulting symptoms are:

- Affect dysregulation
- Dissociation
- Somatic disturbance
- Negative self-image
- Inability to relate and bond to others
- Rupturing of one's belief system

When someone develops PTSD, they keep reliving the event in their minds, and this leads to sensitization and increasing levels of distress with each replay. In replaying the memory of trauma over and over again, a strong neural pathway is created, and it takes less and less stimulation to create a full-blown response as the brain becomes increasingly "wired" in this response. This strong neural pathway is known as a samskara in yoga—feelings and emotions increase in intensity and turn into physical sensations and pain. The body tenses up in protection, thus creating a cycle of tension and pain. One starts to dissociate from the feelings and sensations of the body as the body becomes a living hell. The avoidance of feelings and becoming disconnected from the body is a hallmark trait in PTSD. Essentially, it becomes impossible to experience the present moment. It is important to feel your feelings so that you do not get stuck in them. Feel them out. Let them happen. Then let them go. Otherwise, you may become fixated on the feelings and remain in a constant loop.

Longtime exposure to trauma can leave individuals with feelings of profound shame and worthlessness that affects daily living through the choices they make and how they perceive the world. A body-based therapy plan (yoga) can be highly effective at helping these individuals build resiliency before they begin to explore their traumas with a therapist. A person can heal trauma in the body without ever talking about it. And yoga, specifically, helps to keep the survivor in the present rather than in the trauma of the past.

Somatic and Cognitive Reactions

Somatic and cognitive reactions are normal when we experience overwhelming or traumatic events. It's our body's job to react, and that can sometimes mean life or death. Our bodies give us messages all the time as they pick up information from our senses and send that information to the brain. If we deny or ignore that information, or for some reason can't resolve the incident, then symptoms of trauma occur.

In *Healing Trauma*, author Peter Levine, PhD, breaks down traumatic stress symptoms into three groups, arranged by when they may appear in trauma survivors: immediately, soon after, and prolonged. The following are symptoms that are likely to appear right after the event or soon afterwards:

- Hyperarousal
  - Physical: sweating, increased heart rate, rapid breathing, muscle tension, tingling
  - Mental: racing mind, worry, repetitious thoughts
- Constriction
- Dissociation or denial
- Feelings of helplessness, immobility, and freezing
- Hypervigilance
- Intrusive imagery or flashback
- Extreme sensitivity to light and sound
- Hyperactivity
- Exaggerated emotional and startle responses
- Nightmares and night terrors
- Abrupt mood swings (rage, temper tantrums, frequent anger, crying)
- Shame and lack of self-worth
- Reduced ability to deal with stress
- Difficulty sleeping

Immediately after the event, shock and denial are typical. Longer-term reactions may include unpredictable emotions, flashbacks, strained relationships, and even physical symptoms like headaches or nausea. While these feelings are normal, some people have difficulty moving on with their lives.

The next set of symptoms can show up months or years later if the trauma remains unresolved, including:

- Panic attacks, anxiety, and phobias
- Mental blankness or spaced-out feelings
- Avoidance behavior
- Attraction to dangerous situations
- Addiction
- Change in sexual activity
- Amnesia or forgetfulness
- Inability to bond with others
- Fear of dying
- Self-mutilation
- Loss of sustaining belief system

The final grouping of symptoms, according to Levine, takes longer to develop and may include:

- Excessive shyness
- Diminished emotional responses
- Inability to make commitments
- Chronic fatigue
- Immune system problems
- Psychosomatic illnesses (headache, backache, back problems)
- Chronic pain
- Fibromyalgia
- Asthma
- Skin disorders
- Digestive problems
- Severe PMS (something I have suffered with for years)
- Depression or feeling of impending doom
- Reduced ability to formulate plans

- Compulsion to repeat (re-enactments)

It is important to note that not all of these symptoms will show up in everyone, and there will be various combinations of symptoms as unique as each individual. Sometimes the symptoms are dormant or sometimes they are always present. How do we know if they are due to a trauma? One way is to look at the frequency of occurrence.

Intrusive Symptoms

Intrusive symptoms are those that intrude on the present and are thoughts of the trauma that have the survivor re-experiencing the event: memories in conscious memory; reminders act as triggers; nightmares or distressing dreams can cause a person to relive the experience; flashbacks may cause survivors to think they are in the situation again. Distress is created and defenses are up. As an example, a sexual assault survivor might be driving to work, doing the dishes, or just talking with a friend when suddenly the memory of the sexual assault intrudes on the conscious. These thoughts typically feel like they are out of the blue, they interrupt what the person is doing, and can be extremely upsetting to the person.

A person living with unresolved trauma can re-experience their trauma in a variety of ways. When a person is reminded of the traumatic event, they can experience emotional and physical upset. So as an example, an Iraqi vet may notice that their heart is racing (which would be a physiological reaction) or that they feel fearful (which would be an emotional reaction) when they hear a story on the news about the war. This intrudes on the present moment and the survivor's current state, bringing with it the anxiety and stress of the trauma.

Diagnosing PTSD

To be diagnosed with PTSD, you must have at least three of the five symptoms: avoidance, dissociation, numbing, arousal, and hypervigilance.

Avoidance Symptoms

Because re-experiencing symptoms is so distressing, trauma survivors often work hard to avoid thinking about what happened to them. They will try to avoid thoughts, feelings, or conversations about the event. People with PTSD may turn on the radio, watch television, or just try to keep themselves busy so that they do not have to think about the past event. Unfortunately, studies show that the harder you try not to think about something, the more you actually do think about it; that which we resist, persists.

Another way people practice avoidance is by staying away from activities, places, and people that remind them of the event. A person who has been in a car accident may avoid the site of the accident or might avoid driving on highways if the accident occurred on the highway. A combat veteran may avoid crowds because, in combat situations, crowded places are unsafe. They may choose not to go to restaurants or movies where there are a lot of people and where it may be difficult to escape. A woman who is raped may avoid going to places where there are lots of men such as a bars or clubs, or even grocery stores.

Dissociation Symptoms

Dissociation is a coping mechanism used to create distance between emotions, cognitions, or somatic symptoms. The body becomes a place of hurt. With dissociation, you create compartments for pain, emotions, and memories (explicit memories—a memory without emotional content)—a mental and emotional escape. You may not be able to connect back pain with holding trauma in the body. When you disconnect with pain, you also disconnect with joy, pleasure, and other people. We can't truly connect with others if we cannot connect with ourselves.

Numbing Symptoms

Numbing symptoms prevent the person with PTSD from having intrusive thoughts about what they experienced. Inability to recall part of the trauma refers to a kind of amnesia. It's not due to a head injury, like a car accident victim who hit their head on the steering wheel and can't remember, for example. Rather, these are people who have blocked out an important part of what happened to them when they were traumatized.

People with PTSD find that they also have reduced interest in activities that they used to enjoy. Someone who used to exercise often may find that they are not interested in going to the gym anymore, while someone who used to have a beautiful garden might feel like they have no interest in going out and tending to their yard. This is not about lack of opportunity, it is about a lack of interest, and they just do not feel like it anymore.

Other symptoms include feeling detached from other people, and experiencing a restricted range of emotion. People with PTSD often feel that they are not attached or emotionally close to anybody, that people can't understand them, and that they are emotionally numb.

Arousal Symptoms

To be diagnosed with PTSD, you must have at least two arousal symptoms. Some of these symptoms are similar to what we see in other anxiety disorders such as difficulty sleeping, irritability, or trouble concentrating. It is hard to sleep, stay calm, and keep focused when you are constantly bombarded with intrusive thoughts that get in the way of what you want or need to do.

Hypervigilance Symptoms

People with PTSD tend to be hypervigilant. They are preoccupied with concerns about their own personal safety, or even the safety of loved ones, and are constantly scanning their environment for cues that might signal that danger is around or that they are in a threatening situation. If you were to ask someone with PTSD about their safety cues or their safety routines, they will often say that they are not excessive. However, they tend to go well beyond what most of us do to keep safe. They do not just lock their door at night; instead, they will have an entire routine for checking and making sure that the house is secure. Unfortunately, hypervigilance does not really result in keeping people any safer. It doesn't even result in people being more aware of danger cues. What we see instead is that people with PTSD tend to overreact to safety cues as if they are cues that are signaling danger. They're worried about situations being threatening even though there is no threat present.

Exaggerated Startle Response

The last symptom is an exaggerated startle response. People with PTSD tend to be jumpy and startle easily since they constantly believe they are in a threatening situation.

Coping: Fight—Flight—Freeze

When the coping response to trauma is avoidance or flight, our bodies are preparing to get away from danger and we experience the emotions, anxiety, and fear. The HPA axis (the cross-section of the central nervous system and endocrine system which is responsible for the neuroendocrine adaptation component of the stress response) and the sympathetic nervous system (SNS) activate. Anger and rage combine with SNS and HPA arousal if we are preparing to fight or confront. There is a third option, known as freeze or submit, which appears to activate both the parasympathetic nervous system (PNS) and the SNS. The body is hypervigilant yet immobile. In the animal world, this is seen as "playing dead," and can mean the difference between life and death in some situations. The unmyelinated branch of the vagus nerve is activated, lowering blood pressure and heart rate, and endogenous opiates (natural morphine) are released that blunt pain. In the freeze response, the mind is shut down, and the person is disconnected from the continued real pain the body may be experiencing. The body remembers this pain, and a person with PTSD will suffer from continued somatic expression of this pain in one way or another.

Other Complications of Trauma

When a survivor begins to live with the symptoms of trauma, it becomes difficult to cope. Oftentimes, the coping mechanisms of pre-trauma life no longer work and the survivor begins to take on a new life with new habits. With this, I feel it's imperative to point out a few life-altering complications and behaviors that can occur.

Addiction

If you are suffering from trauma, aside from the obvious propensity for drug and alcohol addiction, even moderate drinking can cause depression. I once had a therapist tell me that if he were to "write a prescription to get depression, he would write alcohol on the script pad." I think about this before I choose to drink and highly advise that you do as well. In states that marijuana is legal, some may find small amounts to be healthier than alcohol. Because marijuana in larger dosages is a psychedelic, however, if you are psychologically unwell or prone to mental illness, I would avoid this altogether. I had a friend who had been diagnosed with bipolar personality disorder and schizophrenia, and once she went from occasional use to daily consumption, she went into a very dark place (and a hospital). I have also seen far too many people who wear their trauma as a badge, try to self-medicate with marijuana, and completely breakdown.

As I mentioned, my own father was medicating himself from combat-related PTSD and drowned himself in a daily sea of martinis. It's hard enough to do your own healing work when sober, the cloud of drugs and alcohol make it almost impossible to see clearly, act with awareness, and make positive, lasting changes. We must be clear to do this work.

An addicted person's impaired ability to stop using drugs and alcohol has to do with deficits in the function of the prefrontal cortex — the part of the brain involved in executive function. The prefrontal cortex has several important jobs: self-monitoring, delaying reward, and integrating whatever the intellect tells you is important. The difficulty also has to do with how the brain, when deprived of the substance to which it is accustomed, reacts to stress. The response is usually exaggerated negative emotion, and even despair. Triggers can include the strong association of learned environmental cues which exacerbate the craving for the substance. The flood of intoxicating brain chemicals called neurotransmitters (chiefly dopamine) during substance use makes the brain change, react, and respond. Again, people with trauma are starting with brains that have been shifted, changed, and damaged because of their traumatic life experiences. The addiction simply becomes an opportunity to escape pain, chase pleasure, and self-medicate.

There are currently active discussions in the addiction and recovery communities around whether or not addiction is truly a disease. In my opinion, this is an important area of discussion. I feel that some people who engage in addiction are already starting with brains that have been affected by trauma or other experiences. The brain changes and develops with repetitive behaviors, and in the addictive process, the person using substances exhibits a repetitive behavior (i.e. drinking every night). Therefore, the brain becomes accustomed to the action. It also changes as a result of the chemical cascade triggered by the substance.

In the DSM V, there are a number of identified substance-use disorders that are defined as diseases. In a state of disease, the part of the body is experiencing physiological abnormalities. I believe addiction can be a learned coping mechanism wherein the brain develops disease from the chemical changes compounded by substances. In a 2018 article from the New England Journal of Medicine titled "Brain Change in Addiction as Learning, Not Disease," Dr. Marc Lewis states that people exposed to trauma are more susceptible to addiction. He says, "Alternatives to the brain-disease model often highlight the social and environmental factors that contribute to addiction, as well as the learning processes that translate these factors into negative outcomes." Dr Lewis concludes that, "exposure to physical, economic, or psychological trauma greatly increases susceptibility to addiction. Learning models propose that addiction, though obviously disadvantageous, is a natural, context-sensitive response to challenging environmental contingencies, not a disease. Yet the brain-disease model construes addictive learning in terms of pathologic brain changes triggered mainly by substance abuse."

An addicted person's impaired ability to stop using drugs and alcohol is contributed to by deficits in the function of the prefrontal cortex—the part of the brain involved in executive function. The prefrontal cortex has several important jobs: self-monitoring, delaying reward, and integrating whatever the intellect tells you is important. The difficulty also has to do with how the brain, when deprived of the substance to which it is accustomed, reacts to stress. The response is usually exaggerated negative emotion and even despair. Triggers can include the strong association of learned environmental cues which exacerbate the craving for the substance. The flood of intoxicating brain chemicals called neurotransmitters (including dopamine, which modulates our motivation and reward pathways) influences how the brain changes, reacts, and responds. People with trauma in their history may also be experiencing dysregulation from changes in brain function resulting from their traumatic life experiences. Addiction becomes an opportunity to escape pain, chase pleasure, and self-medicate. No matter the drug or behavior of choice, the cycle of addiction includes seeking methods of self-medicating and self-soothing.

No matter what the drug of choice is, addiction simply becomes a method of medicating and self-soothing. I know too many people dependent on carbs, sugar, and shopping, not to mention more intoxicating substances. While trauma may drive some of us to addiction, we are starting with a brain that is already damaged and then the addiction creates more damage.

How Healing Happens

Bessel A. van der Kolk, in his book *The Body Keeps Score*, says that emotional pain and traumatic memories can be stored in the body long after exposure. He promotes somatic treatment for trauma and PTSD. He points out that, when traumatized people try to talk about the trauma, they shut down due to feelings of helplessness, fear, shame, and rage overwhelming them when memories surface.

However, even when the impact on the brain seems overwhelming and difficult to comprehend, the healing process is possible. The changes to the brain during trauma are substantial, but can be reversed with the attention and self-care that it needs. The amygdala can transition back to calm and relaxed; the hippocampus can once again maintain memory consolidation; the nervous system can balance between reactive and restorative modes. A proactive effort to rebalance the body and mind is the key to healing.

The body and mind can recalibrate through exercises and activities specifically designed to focus on tension release, such as yoga. But as each trauma experience is unique to the individual, so is the healing process. With time and dedication, the symptoms of PTSD can be drastically alleviated, if not eliminated completely.

Survivor story: Greg

If, prior to the fall of 2018, you were to ask me what kind of childhood I had, I probably would have responded that it was tough, but we survived. Through my YogaFit training I now understand that my upbringing was, from a child's perspective, somewhat of a traumatic one. One that was filled with anxiety and lacked consistent emotional parental support. It is no wonder that at thirteen years old I started drinking alcohol, and just a few years later in high school, I added drugs to my toxic coping mix. It is also no surprise that, directly from high school, I decided to join the military. At the tender age of seventeen, the military raised me. This decision was one of bravery and courage as I had two great uncles who served in World War II. I do not have any regrets. I would do it all over again. True, it was something I wanted to pursue and was excited about, but I now understand that in a sense, I was running from, and for, my life.

On December 12th, 1985, my life changed. Just two weeks before Christmas, Arrow Air Flight 1285 with members of the 101st Airborne Division out of Fort Campbell, Kentucky, was returning home from a deployment in the Sinai. It landed in Gander, Newfoundland where I was stationed, and crashed shortly after taking off. 248 soldiers and eight crew members were lost. 256 souls — perished. We were sent in to do recovery. What I witnessed was nothing short of what I imagined a battlefield of one of the Great Wars would have been like. The experience left me feeling numb, heartbroken, and helpless. It was as if my soul had stepped outside of my physical body.

A 34-year career in the service certainly took its toll. Military training in itself always has our bodies constantly in a high state of readiness; ready for fight or flight. Any and every deployment that I was on, domestic or otherwise was an intense stressor. I frequently flashed back to Gander and always seemed to be in a highly hyper-vigilant state. If only the military included a trauma-preventative yoga practice in our training. A practice that helps guide our bodies back from potentially traumatic or highly stressful situations. If only the training included effective yogic methods that allowed us to de-stress from the psychological austerity associated with being deployed. My coping strategies included alcohol, being entrenched in my work, and running—anything that would deflect my mind from the horrors hidden deep inside it. If only we were taught how to practice *Dhyana, Pranayama,* and *Asana.* Yoga poses and breathing techniques that activated and stimulated our parasympathetic and vagus nervous systems. How resilient a soldier could be if only these tools were in their rucksack. If only.

When I retired, the trauma I experienced came back. It came back with vengeance. Nightmares returned with a deepened intensity and my flashbacks were more frequent. Everything seemed to trigger me. I didn't feel safe to go anywhere. Emotionally void and detached from myself and those who loved me, I slowly slipped into a deep, dark, demonic hole where my only solution was to drink. I was depressed, anxious, and suicidal. I was one drink away from carrying out my plan to kill myself.

I am fortunate to have a loving, supportive family. It was during this all-time low in my life when my current spouse had the courage to sit me down at the kitchen table and express her concern for me. I guess, subconsciously, having someone express love and compassion for me was what gave me the courage to tell her I was planning on hurting myself. At the time I couldn't even say the word suicide. The stigma around mental health is so powerful and debilitating — it is sometimes fatal. If not for her loving response, I'm not sure how my story would have ended. That day at the kitchen table, she held me for what seemed like an eternity, as I wept like an infant in her embrace.

In 2014 I was diagnosed with PTSD and started practicing yoga. I didn't know what it was about yoga, but I knew it was helping. I remember a session with my psychologist who challenged me and asked what it was about yoga that I was finding helpful. My response was that it grounds me and reconnects me with my body. It didn't make sense to me then, but thanks to my training through YogaFit, it does now. How we disconnect from our bodies in an attempt to survive; how our bodies need to recover and bounce back from a fight and flight response. I am so grateful for yoga and the unification it has given me with my mind, body, and soul. The acceptance of who I am and the contentment it brings and the space it creates within me. I am grateful for the teachings of Ayurveda; and how, coupled with yoga, it can help me find physical and spiritual centering.

PTSD is a very terrifying affliction. It consumes me. My injured nervous system and brain has me sometimes processing information in a far more hyper-aroused rate. This can be detrimental. It is mentally exhausting. I recall one instance in the hospital emergency room where what seemed to be a lapse in my ability to control my anxiety had me terrified and very aggressive. So much so, I was eventually restrained by the wrists and ankles and chained to the floor in the treatment room. I don't remember much after the sedation, but it was then I started being medicated for my illness. I tried several medications that either made my symptoms worse or caused adverse physical side effects. I am currently taking a medication for depression, albeit at a low dose which I attribute to yoga, which I do find helpful. My goal is that through my yoga practice there will be no need for me to take any pharmaceuticals to treat my PTSD.

In 2015 I took part in a transition program hosted by the Veteran's Transition Network. During the program we talked about setting long term goals. One of mine was to someday teach yoga to fellow veterans whom have been nightmarishly afflicted with PTSD. In the spring of 2018 I decided I was ready to start this journey.

After sometime of searching online, the Warrior Program offered by YogaFit caught my eye. In October 2018 I completed the Level One Foundations training. I was immediately drawn into YogaFit and their disciplines. The essence of yoga, I believe, is also the essence of recovering from trauma. It was apparent to me that YogaFit had done their homework and had many highly informed and compassionate people delivering the courses. I was so inspired that I decided that this was where I wanted to deepen my practice and train to become a yoga instructor.

As my training progressed, it all started to come together: why certain poses worked for me and why others didn't; why some essential oils might ground and calm me, and why others may be triggering me; why the characteristic of some yoga teachers and their instructional technique triggered me and had me thinking that I would probably not return to their class, or conversely, had me loving their class and had me excited about returning the following week.

Why was I drawn to a yinful and restorative practice but also in love with vinyasa. I thoroughly enjoy a vinyasa class that consists of a therapeutic flowing sequence, of slow and deliberative movement. It is a class that also includes choice. I always seem to leave these practices feeling connected, invigorated, and in control. Yoga nidra is also something I try to practice at least once a month. I have attained levels of meditation and connection to my body during nidra which I have not been able to attain in any other practice.

I believe that transformational language and positive affirmation are fundamentally the building blocks for a trauma informed yoga class. I find it fosters a safe and inclusive environment, promotes trust, and helps keep me present—all very significant barriers for a trauma survivor to overcome. Trauma certainly holds no prejudices and does not discriminate. It kidnaps bodies of all ages and is a cancer to our true self. It is not exclusive to military personnel and first responders. I feel that a trauma-informed instructor understands that at any time any student who has experienced trauma, could be instantaneously triggered and reliving that terrifying moment. Perhaps it is a smell, a sound, or a touch. Perhaps it is a pose. Maybe it is nothing. Flashbacks are like a heinous intruder that seems to stalk us and enter our minds without warning. They paralyze the mind and body, creating a state of panic that shuts us down.

To this day, given the right conditions, I can experience an unprovoked flashback. Savasana seems to be my most challenging pose and the one I have come to love. Whether it is the temperature of the room or the pounding of my heart because I have just finished a very energetic flow practice, I am instantaneously re-living a traumatic event. My body remembers. It does not forget. It is my yoga practice that rescues me when these events occur. I only need to remind myself to return to my breath and repeat my mantra: I am safe, I am laying on my mat in *Savasana*, practicing Hatha Yoga.

Satya — Truthfulness: the second of the five *Yamas* is my steel. When I struggle, and I often do, I always return to *Satya*. For, if I am true to myself, I am true to my practice. If I am true to my practice, I am true to me and everyone and everything that surrounds me. One of the greatest joys that yoga has given me is the reconnection to my emotions; a connection to the loving, nurturing man that society and the experiences I have had while serving has tried to suppress.

Yoga has given me the tools I need to lead a healthier and more productive life. It reduces my stress and has me loving myself again. It is a resource I can turn to at any time. It grounds me and reconnects me with my body. YogaFit is giving me the confidence, knowledge, and tools I need to deliver a loving, trauma-informed class. With it I hope to fulfill my goal and return life to the faces of those suffering from trauma.

Yoga reconnects me to my inner child—that fearless, playful, silly, and loving little boy, who adored nature and every living organism in it. That resilient inner child who I believe is the bridge to our true self.

Yoga gives me a profound connection to a divine spirituality that resides within me. It resides within each and every one of us. It is a spirituality of love and kindness. It is one that is never-ending and one that perseveres. It is a spirituality that has nowhere to go but out.

CHAPTER 2

The Power of Yoga

"No effort on the yoga path is ever lost, nor can any obstacle ever hold one back forever. Just a little progress on this path can protect one from the greatest fear."

—BHAGAVAD GITA 2:40

History of Yoga

Yoga is commonly known to be over 6,000 years and has a very storied past. Yoga combines a wealth of practices that build a better body and a stronger mind using physical movement, breath control, and meditative focus. Physical yoga, *asana*, was designed to prepare the body for meditation. There are tales of yogis performing miraculous feats of the body. According to the third book of the *Sutras*, if one dedicated themselves to the practice of yoga, it was said, they would obtain *siddhis*, or supernatural powers. There are stories of yoga masters slowing down their hearts, having psychic powers, and living for hundreds of years. Over time, yoga became a system of psychological and physical practices to create greater health, mental awareness, and balance. My own first formal yoga teacher healed her cancer through yoga. From its earliest introduction, people have known yoga's power to heal, calm the mind, and promote peace.

Trauma survivors have a loss of power and control and feel as if they are not safe in their own bodies. There is disconnection and distrust of the body, the mind, and the world around them. Anxiety and depression result, and coping strategies may include alcohol, drugs (including prescription), or other addictions. Healing and moving past trauma requires that a survivor find ways to restore a sense of control to their lives. Yoga can be a life-saving tool and can help a trauma survivor to find a joyful life again.

Different forms and techniques evolved; at YogaFit and in this book, we teach the "hatha yoga tradition of the *vinyasa* style." Yoga, in its most simple meaning, means union. Hatha yoga, which is the physical portion of the practice, means to unite the sun and the moon, to bring together in unison all duality and aspects of the self. Hatha derives from the thirteenth-century Sanskrit and means several things. It literally translates to "force" or "physical," but it can be poetically broken down into "ha" and "tha." Ha represents the qualities of masculine, solar, or energizing; Tha represents the qualities of feminine, lunar, or relaxing. The word hatha invokes the balance of opposites. This lends itself to my belief that the practice of yoga is the yin (healing) to the yang (trauma), and that, somehow through this joining, we form a stronger self. In my own experience, had I not experienced trauma as a child, I may not have had the opportunity, the pull, and the inclination towards the healing that yoga brings. Fortunately, my healing process has created a vehicle in which many others can be and have been healed. YogaFit is this vehicle. Healing is an ongoing, one-day-at-a-time process.

Yoga is a science of mind that can be used to understand, accept, and shift the mind-body. I like to say that "yoga meets you where you are, whenever and wherever you are." Yoga is a safe haven for all.

Ancient yoga practitioners used the system of hatha yoga as preparation for long periods of sitting. Many people "sit" with trauma; I frequently say when I teach classes that "yoga allows us the opportunity to get comfortable being uncomfortable." If we cannot "heal our trauma," we can at least learn to sit with it comfortably and mitigate the associated symptoms with our practice of mindfulness and the heightened levels of consciousness that our practice brings. Yoga itself is the union of opposites. For me that means that I can experience immense pain and sadness, but also abundant joy and peace. In non-dualistic thinking, we accept the totality of what is, what we are, and what we can transform ourselves into. I believe that yoga transforms us every single time we practice.

Much of what is presented as yoga in the west is *asana*, the physical poses. While these are potent and transformative, *asana* (the postures), are just one of the many tools yoga has for healing. Yes, *asana* is, in part, physical exercise, but it also works with the gross and subtle body. It makes us strong and flexible, awakens our energy centers, opens our channels, and helps us focus the mind with the breath. The eight limbs of yoga provide us a goal of self-realization and enlightenment, creating an environment for optimal physical and mental health. While yoga helps me maintain a consistent state of physical, mental, and emotional health consciousness I am.

The eight-limbed path of the yoga lifestyle is a guide to finding stillness of the mind. In that peace and stillness, we find a connection to the divine or the present moment and enlightenment. Think of it like a roadmap that helps guide us through our life path. The eight limbs provide a way for the trauma survivor to become centered and grounded and reconnect with the strengths and resources that are available in each person. To move past trauma, the survivor needs to learn to befriend the body because the mind and body are strongly intertwined. And with the impact of trauma, both are greatly affected.

In yoga, we learn that if we can find contentment and focus on the present moment, we will find joy. Trauma survivors can lose this connection to the present moment and, as a result, can easily lose their sense of peace, joy, and connection to others.

The Eight Limbs of Healing Trauma

Through yoga, the goal is to become connected physically, mentally, and spiritually. These are the traditional limbs of yoga to help you better understand how following the path of these limbs will help you lead a clearer and more connected life.

I find that, if I feel off course, the eight limbs of yoga help get me back on track. They are great reminders of how I want to personally live. They truly inspire and motivate me.

These are the eight limbs of yoga and how they relate to trauma and the daily healing process.

Yamas and Niyamas

1. *Yamas:* the physical principles that involve speaking, eating, and breathing in a way to lead to living your best life.

   - *Ahimsa:* non-violence and inflicting no injury or harm to others and one's own self. It also asks that we restrain from violence in thought, word, and deed; the practice of nonviolence toward us and other living beings. This applies to practicing nonviolence with our thoughts and actions. For those who are victims of trauma and had violence forced upon them, *ahimsa* may be very hard to practice because we want to continue to perpetrate violence to others and ourselves. This violence may come from a desire to exact revenge or because we are so hurt and angry at the world. As recipients of trauma, we may become conditioned to keep seeking it because this becomes our norm and a state in which we have learned to function. We many become critical to ourselves in words and action and turn the violence inward. Many times, this results in self-sabotage, self-harm, and criticism. This is a time when addiction can easily enter the picture.

   - *Satya:* non-illusion and remaining true in our words and thoughts; the practice of honesty in speech, thoughts, and deeds, always with the intention to heal or help, not hurt. This is both outwards and inwards, truthful with ourselves and truthful with others. Often, when there is trauma, there is shame; where there is shame, there is deceit or denial. Our goal with *satya* is to be more truthful and more transparent. "We are only as sick as the secrets we keep," comes from Alcoholics Anonymous. We can use *satya*, the policy of truth, to help ourselves heal.

   - *Asteya:* to not covet things in other's possession and our own; the practice of taking what only belongs to us—discerning and seeking only what we need versus what we want. I believe this also means "non-coveting." We shouldn't desire what seems to be someone else's picture perfect life, their "trauma-free" childhood, or what may seem like someone else's easy life. Take what belongs to us; suffering from trauma, depression, and PTSD does not mean we get to "steal someone else's joy." Nor does it mean we need to steal our own joy, our own heart's desires, or our own lives. Also, we shouldn't let anyone steal our peace, our joy, our calm, or our life. This includes those who may have caused our trauma—we do not give them the privilege of stealing our lives!

- *Brahmacharya:* abstinence and using our energy to move forward in our goal of reaching the truth, suggesting that our relationships that foster our understanding of the highest truths; the practice of moderation in all areas of life, from food consumption and exercise to sleep and work. Many times when a trauma is experienced, we may want to overindulge in alcohol, drugs, food, sex, shopping, partying, gambling, working, or exercise. I know my own addictions come in the form of exercise, love addiction, and work. Learn to be still and practice "having less to BE more." Moderation means to be balanced and calm in our desires.

- *Aparigraha:* non-possessiveness; non-hoarding; the practice of letting go of all worldly, extraneous items and relationships that we rely on for our peace and happiness or non-attachment to the material world. We may have built a fortress around ourselves because of trauma. The walls many be made of different things for different people—weight, possessions, clutter, stuff, money. By letting go of those things that may be blocking our healing, we knock down the walls and heal.

2. *Niyamas:* the five observances: how we relate to ourselves, the inner world. The *niyamas* are guidelines for how we interact with ourselves and our internal world. The practice of the *niyamas* harnesses the energy created through the practice and application of the *yamas*. While these principles are about our inner life, their impact will reach far beyond ourselves.

- *Saucha:* cleanliness of body and mind. Our body is a temple and needs to be treated as such. This is the practice of keeping our temple clean and free of toxins: people, places, substances, and habits that do not serve us. Where our environment is clean and clear, when our body is free of mind altering or unhealthy things, we will feel better. For those of us recovering from trauma and trying to keep our "stuff" together, the practice of simple cleanliness goes a very long way in navigating life from a centered place. I find *saucha* especially beneficial and strive towards a clean interior and exterior daily. Let *saucha* become your daily practice.

- *Santosha:* satisfaction with what one already has; the practice of contentment. Just being happy about our progress on a healing path is *santosha*. Doing something good for ourselves every day will help us feel content with who we are, what we have, and our journey this far. Celebrate the small victories and keep a state of gratitude that leads to being more content. I find the simple practice of gratitude keeps me lifted out of my trauma-based darkness. Many of my spiritual advisers (healers, spiritual coaches) recently encouraged me to make peace with my father. I was at jazz music festival while finishing this book, and I remembered his love of music and how that had been imparted unto me, and I was grateful. I was also reminded to focus on the positives. Gratitude goes a long way in healing.

- *Tapas:* austerity and associated observances for body discipline and thereby mental control; the practice of discipline. Because having trauma, PTSD, depression, or anxiety can force us to feel like giving in, giving up, and picking up unhealthy habits, we must rigorously practice healthy things that make us feel good and are good for us. Attending a twelve-step meeting, exercising, eating well, resting, and taking care of ourselves all require discipline. Just like training for a marathon, we have to run. Losing weight requires discipline. Discipline begets and creates more discipline. Order creates order. Use your fire, however it was started, to light a bigger fire—and burn up in the flames of healing.

- *Svādhyāya:* study of the Vedic scriptures to know about God and the soul, which leads to introspection on a greater awakening to the soul and God within; the practice of self-observation. Becoming the witness to our body, emotions, and mind. Use the Essence of YogaFit—no judgement, no expectation, no competition—when you observe yourself. Be gentle but firm, like a good parent. Many of us who had absentee parents and have experienced trauma will have to actually learn to "reparent" ourselves. Hold that sacred little child, the traumatized teenager or our depressed younger self in your arms and in our heart. *Svādhyāya* allows us to show up for ourselves, observe, be the ever present witness even when we may have felt unseen and then course-correct as needed to be our best selves. *Svādhyāya* can be summed up in one word: mindfulness. The path of self-education and study comes through internal awareness and external resources— Cognitive Behavioral Therapy (CBT) is based on mindfulness. Yoga and meditation give us mindfulness. Therapy one-on-one or in a group brings us a reflection by which we can see ourselves more accurately. By learning to step back and breathe, we will better understand our own reactions, and what triggers them, which will help us become aware (and conscious) about how we are treating ourselves.

- *Ishvara pranidhana:* surrender, the practice of surrender. Surrender to what is and what was. What happened, happened. The AA Serenity Prayer is "God grant me the serenity to accept the things I cannot change, the courage to change the things I can, and the wisdom to know the difference." Through the practices of yoga, we will slowly begin to unclench trauma from our bodies, minds, and spirits. Peace, calm, and joy may follow.

3. *Asana:* physical postures creating awareness and self-discipline of the body through yoga poses. We learn to take care of our physical structure through *asana*.

4. *Pranayama:* breath work. We regulate and control life force energies through breathing. We connect the body and mind with intentional breathing practices.

5. *Pratyahara:* self-study to be the witness to the mind-body. We can then take an honest look at ourselves and objectively observe our growth, progress, and our need to refine.

6. *Dharana:* concentration, one pointed focus. We practice by choosing one thing to focus on and practice this important and often-absent skill. The best place to start practicing this is in yoga class—focus on the body and focus on your breath.

7. *Dhyana:* meditation, the ability to both free and control the mind and, at the same time, let go of expectations to do either.

8. *Samadhi:* bliss, oneness, transcendence beyond the earth plane, connection to all cosmic consciousness and oneness. Become one with the universe and achieve a state of natural ecstasy with ease and with bliss.

The eight limbs of yoga teach skills and habits needed to heal and become whole. They provide a guideline from which to live and provide goals for us to become closer to the universe, all consciousness, and ourselves. The greatest opportunity for total transformation is to become fully present to yourself, your life's purpose, and your infinite potential.

In the following chapters we will discover how to maneuver, develop, and practice limbs of:

- *Pranayama:* Breathing
- *Asana:* Yoga poses
- *Dhyana:* Meditation
- *Pratyahara:* Study of self
- *Dharana:* Concentration
- *Samadhi:* Living our best lives

Traditionally, these limbs were studied in order. So before anyone studied the physical postures, they are expected to adhere to the ethical rules and restraints. And, it makes sense. Yoga is a powerful tool of healing and transformation and, "With great power, comes great responsibility." We get what we put out; like is attracted to like. So, if we're lying or stealing, we probably won't be too successful in hearing our voices and healing our bodies.

When you are able to get yoga as more than just exercise or doing poses, then you start to understand through deep feeling the power of yoga's therapeutic applications. Yoga has been used in conjunction with Ayurveda for the purpose of total mind-body healing since its inception. Yoga is natural and organic.

You may wonder, what is yoga therapy? It is using the totality of physical postures, breath work, and meditation to heal. While all yoga poses are healing, but yoga therapy is a systematic approach to specific ailments using a variety of yoga practices. It uses gentle *asana, pranayama,* meditation, visualization, and diet. I am a yogi; I put great importance on what I put in my body. Foods either heal, are neutral, or harm; certain foods and drinks can agitate one's mind, and some will calm the nerves. In my book *YogaLean,* I discuss the concept of lean consciousness, being able to look at a food or beverage and feel how it will make you feel. This gives you the choice in whether or not to ingest it. We can actually learn to feel the vibration, the energy, and the contents of something in a way that gives us the power of choice.

To help understand the power and strength of yoga as a tool for healing trauma, it is useful to understand yoga anatomy. Much like Chinese meridians in acupuncture, yogis have *nadis*. There are 72,000 psychic channels, or *nadis*, circulating *prana* throughout our bodies. *Prana* is the life force, similar to *chi* in Chinese medicine. These *nadis* can have knots, or *granthis*, that need to be removed for the flow of *prana* to move freely through the body and our consciousness to rise. Interestingly, yogis believe that, where there is tightness in our body, the *prana* is stuck there.

According to yoga anatomy, we have five *koshas*, or layers, and pain or illness can sprout from trauma to any of these *koshas*. The koshas go from the gross body to the subtle body, and all of the *koshas* have a great effect on one's well-being and health. The five *koshas* are:

1. *Anamaya:* The physical body; muscle, bones, organs, etc.
2. *Pranamaya:* The subtle body; breath, prana, etc.
3. *Manomaya:* Thoughts and emotions
4. *Vijnanamaya:* Intuition and knowledge
5. *Anandamaya:* Bliss

If something is wrong in any one of these layers, illness and disease will be the result. For example, if someone is working a toxic environment, then it is quite likely that they will get sick. The yoga therapist will look at the person's life holistically and prescribe exercises to heal them. By using *asana, pranayama,* meditation, and other powerful techniques, one is able to heal the body.

For many trauma victims, their coping mechanism is to block all sensations in the body. They tend to not live in their bodies and don't feel much of anything. Yoga therapy helps them live and feel their bodies. For many victims of trauma, the lasting effect isn't the actual event, it's what they can't let go of. In yoga this is called a *samskara*, and it is imprints of past traumas or negative karmas that we carry with us. Yogis look at the person holistically and heal the body, mind, and spirit.

It's challenging to have perfect health in the body if the mind or spirit is injured. Through postures, breathing techniques, and meditations, one is able to bring the body back into balance. While completely erasing the trauma might not be possible, yoga can help heal the resulting disorders.

Trauma affects more than one *kosha*, and to be able to treat the trauma, a holistic treatment needs to be implemented. The survivor of trauma must learn to live in their body and release the trauma's effects on the body, mind, and spirit. Dr. Bessel van der Kolk presented findings in 2010 to the International Society for Traumatic Stress Studies conference. He found in the initial studies that there was a thirty percent reduction in symptoms of posttraumatic stress for a participant of trauma-informed gentle yoga after only ten-weeks.[5]

These are remarkable results in just a short time and illustrate once more the tremendous power and scope of the science of yoga. Yoga is a powerful tool for healing and has been for thousands of years.

"Trauma-Sensitive Yoga" is a term coined by David Emerson, E-RYT, founder and director at the Trauma Center at the Justice Resource Institute in Brookline, Massachusetts. It is a practice that uses modified yoga techniques to support clinical treatment and help patients feel comfortable in their bodies again, foster self-awareness and regulation, increase resiliency, and become present in order to reconnect with daily life and relationships.

Yoga gives us that space, and trauma-sensitive yoga helps victims of trauma reenter their bodies and find that peace and relaxation.

A smaller study showed that yoga increases heart rate variability (HRV), a measurement for how strong the brain's arousal system is. For trauma victims, the HRV is abnormally low. Dr. van der Kolk believes this is why traumatized people are more prone to illness and stress. "Yoga's ability to touch us on every level of our being—physical, mental, emotional, and spiritual—makes it a powerful and effective means for trauma victims to reinhabit their bodies safely, calm their minds, experience emotions directly, and begin to feel a sense of strength and control." Yoga works on many levels, and once we can see the body and the layers of *koshas* and thousands of *nadis*, we can begin to grasp the magnitude and power of yoga.

Over half the population has experienced at least one traumatic event, and five percent of men and ten percent of women have developed PTSD. [6] I believe these statistics are vastly underreported. People with PTSD have a hard time calming down or self-regulating and have a lower HRV. Seventy-

5   *Yoga International Transcending Trauma: How Yoga Heals*
6   Trauma-Sensitive Yoga: Principles, Practice, and Research. David Emerson, E-RYT, Ritu Sharma, PHD, Serena Chaudhry, Jen Turner

four percent of people diagnosed with PTSD have symptoms for more than six months, with some being symptomatic throughout their life. According to the US National Comorbidity Survey, eighty-eight percent of people with PTSD have a higher chance of other psychiatric illness, and, according to an Australian study, women with PTSD were twenty-three times more likely to develop depression, ten times more likely to develop anxiety disorders, and ten times more likely to have panic disorders.[7]

Beyond the healing effects of many yoga postures, there are many mind-body practices to calm the mind and balance the nervous system. It's not one-stop shopping; not all techniques are applicable to all diseases. While some practices may be beneficial to lowering blood pressure, others will be used for anxiety or to combat the symptoms of menopause or, yes, alleviate the symptoms of PTSD.

Yoga is powerful—an ancient practice designed for ultimate health and vitality on every level—and it works. Yoga continues to grow in popularity for those suffering from trauma and PTSD because it offers a respite through its poses and techniques that enhances the physical, mental, emotional, and energetic aspects. The mindfulness learned fosters a stable emotional being and reduces tension and fatigue.

As the study and practice of yoga for trauma expands and deepens, we see its many proven successes in the treatment and relief from many symptoms of trauma. We have a hard time healing our bodies when we can't inhabit them. After we have spent years numbing the pain from trauma, it is hard to inhabit one's body again. Yoga makes that journey possible and, yoga holds a safe place for us all.

The Essence of YogaFit

In our YogaFit trainings, we teach the Essence of YogaFit to enthusiast, novice, teacher, and practitioner to help them relate to themselves and their students. The seven steps assist us in staying present in the moment and remind us to have grace while listening to our bodies. This process allows us to move through our feelings, staying connected to ourselves.

---

7   *Trauma Sensitive Yoga: Principles, Practice, and Research.* David Emerson, E-RYT; Ritu Sharma PhD; Serena Chaudhry; Jen Turner.

The Essence of YogaFit guides us mentally and psychologically through our practice allowing us to stay on our path of healing.

1. **Breathing**—the breath is our most powerful tool to relax our bodies and clear our minds. Breathing also allows us to regroup and stay present. Taking a minute to gather yourself with deep breaths will refocus your entire being. Life is fast-paced, and if we give ourselves the space to close our eyes and inhale deeply, filling our body with good thoughts and intentions while slowly exhaling the negative, we will stay on track. I constantly have to remind myself to breathe.

2. **Feeling**—we want to feel something in every pose, action, and thought. In yoga, we are always reminded to check in with our bodies in order to modify poses to provide less or more sensation. When we feel something in our bodies, we stay grounded in the moment and in awareness of our body and its potential. Learning to accept and work with your feelings will give you a better sense of how to shift those feelings from negative to positive.

3. **Listening to our bodies**—our body tells us everything we need to know. The trick is learning to listen to your body when it whispers because if you don't it will break down and become a roar. Yoga teaches us to listen to our body through presence, awareness, and witness consciousness.

4. **Letting Go of Competition**—our bodies are like snowflakes; everyone is unique based on genetics and life experiences. I know many times I have felt that life is not fair, and my mind may say, "Why couldn't I have grown up in a happy, supportive, non-traumatic house." Then I realize that by letting go of competition, allowing for my own unique healing journey, and not comparing or competing with others, I stay grounded on my own path.

5. **Letting Go of Judgment**—it is important to let go of judgment if you have a challenging day or on any day. Many times if we have suffered trauma, have PTSD or been given a psychological diagnosis (a label like acute depression, bipolar, PTSD, mania,), we may harshly judge ourselves. Words like "damaged," "crazy," and "ruined" may become part of our self-identity, which is why I'm not particularly a fan of labels. We may judge or blame ourselves for the experience or our

reaction to it by thinking, "Why can't I just get over this?" However, by letting go of judgement we are able to simply BE. We forgive ourselves when we let go of judgement. This forgiveness helps us heal.

6. **Letting Go of Expectations**—in yoga, we turn our attention inward. Encouraging ourselves to let go of external comparisons and judgments allows us to have a deeper experience in our Yoga practice. We learn to let go of competition and expectations; we practice based on how we feel today, not how we felt in our last yoga class. Yoga is a process and a journey, not a destination. By letting go of expecting that we should "be" a certain way, "healed" in a certain time frame, or "over" our trauma, we practice acceptance and show up for ourselves.

7. **Staying in the Present Moment**

   In yoga we are taught that, if we can find contentment and focus on the present moment, we will find joy. Trauma survivors have lost this connection to the present moment and, as a result, have lost their sense of peace, joy, and connection to others. By asking yourself, "How am I in this moment?" we clear away a lot of the past having an effect on our present. Chances are that we are doing in ok in the moment, if we can just stay present.

Survivor story: **Debbie**

My husband and I adopted and raised two children who ended up getting into drugs. Despite our best efforts, we could not turn the tide of their decisions and, as they headed into their late teens, they both became very aggressive and threatening. My husband and I eventually made the tough decision to move far away from them. By the time they were old enough to live on their own, I was having panic and anxiety attacks and was terrified much of the time. I thought there was something terribly wrong with me and that I would never be happy.

Knowing that I needed to do something to make a change, I began to practice shamatha (resting or calm abiding) meditation as taught to me by a seasoned practitioner and Tibetan Buddhist monk in Memphis, TN. Specifically, he taught me to attend at the start of meditation to three things: body, breath and mind.

1. Body—sit the body safely and comfortably by keeping spine straight, crossing legs, palms on thighs; heart open; chin humbled slightly toward the chest; tongue lightly placed on palette behind the top teeth; breathe through mouth, nose, or both; eyes open especially if the mind is sleepy, but eyes closed if the mind is busy to close off some sources of stimulation. One can meditate anywhere, at any time, in any position, including laying down, as long as the body can be comfortable, safe, and relaxed. Position the body so it can be stable and doesn't fall over if seated or fall asleep if lying down.

2. Breath—take a few deep breaths then breathe normally. It is very important to relax deeply with every exhalation.

3. Mind—the most important aspect. Place the attention on the breath, following it in and following it out. When the mind wanders, just notice, let the thought go, and gently and kindly bring attention back to the breath. When thoughts come, just know it is the normal function of the mind. However, don't "think the thoughts," e.g., during meditation, if the thought "I am hungry" arises, just let the thought go and don't continue on by thinking, "I think there is some cold pizza and salad at home. Well, I'd rather have some hummus so I'll have to go to the store." Also, there is no need to push thoughts away because they dissolve on their own if one doesn't hang on to them.

Eventually my mind began to calm down and rest. By doing this practice, I began to "see" and "hear" that the scary thoughts or mental movies that caused me such anguish were just that—thoughts. Some were stressful memories from the past or the expectation of possible (and imaginary) discomfort that might happen in the future, but NONE existed in the present moment. I was feeling anxious in the present moment over something imaginary!

As I began to understand through meditation how the mind presents stories that don't exist right now, I began to be able to place space between the thought and my reaction to it. This allowed me to be better able to choose how to react. I started noticing how certain stories were precursors to pains or discomfort in my body. I could also let the stories go and prevent the pains with what I was learning about the mind in meditation.

I practiced staying present and being mindful of what was happening in the mind and also what was happening in the present moment in life. By doing this, I began to notice the many small things going on around me constantly that can bring joy—the beautiful colors of the grass in my yard, the sound of birds, the warmth and scent of freshly laundered and dried clothing, the taste of my food. I practiced staying present for all the joyful things around me. This practice continually helps me to keep a joyful mind, and has eliminated a lot of the mental negativity I had developed as a bad and harmful habit.

As a byproduct, people around me seemed to change. People I'd had problems with seemed to become more enjoyable, even "nicer," and the people in my circle of friends and acquaintances became less troubled and happier. Meditation truly is magic!

As you can imagine, the stress on our marriage was enormous. As I calmed myself and responded better to our children's situations, the relationship with my husband improved greatly.

As I continued to practice meditation and mindfulness, I began to notice that some of the food I ate actually made me feel bad in the body. Meat made me feel sluggish, sweets after dinner gave me a sugar rush that contributed to restless leg syndrome and middle-of-the-night heartburn, and eating too much actually hurt my back when I meditated or had to stand for long periods at work. So I began to experiment with food and what and when I ate. When I began to do yoga, I began seeing further how foods affected my physical strength and stamina. In an effort to feel better physically and practice non-harming, I stopped eating meat and cut back sugar to almost none. I feel much better.

There came a point about eight months ago when I got some disturbing news from my doctor about some blood tests. I further revised my food intake by doing research and adding in foods valued to bring certain benefits, and I became more regular about doing different breathing techniques. I can actually see the calming results of doing these practices on my fitness app when I do them for even short periods of time. They basically calm me within a minute. I knew pranayama can be purifying and healing, so I did it often. Within about five weeks, the issues in my bloodwork resolved.

My meditation practice also led to a change in my consumption patterns. I noticed that the unending desire for some new material possession was also fueling a need for more money, resulting in needing to work more hours. I began to really examine whether or not I really needed it every time I went to buy something. Now when I go shopping, I often come home empty-handed. With mindful consumption, I have cut back spending and have been able to retire and devote my time to what I deem to be important.

Last but not least is my yoga practice. I perform it as a moving meditation, watching my mind as I move and breathe, and identifying many of the same habitual patterns that I experience in my day-to-day life. The yoga has helped me ease the tension I hold in my muscles, organs, and joints. I see the results of my mental patterns in my body, and I work to let those patterns go so I can be more comfortable and relaxed. I am a work in progress, but it is fascinating, worthwhile, and rewarding work that I will do for the rest of my life (I am sixty-two!) and I will teach others whatever I can to help for as long as I am able.

So, you can see that in a big way, meditation and mindfulness is the thing that informed and changed many areas throughout my life and has ultimately led to being happier. Having a knowledgeable and experienced meditation teacher has been an indispensable asset. My teacher has always been someone who would answer my questions, and someone who could give me a reasoned response from a meditative perspective about the goings-on in my life. Now, my life is by no means perfect; many areas still have ongoing or periodic problems, but my response to these problems has changed and my mental attitude is healthier. That mental change has made all the difference!

I had started to meditate, and once we moved, I found a wonderful meditation teacher and began to really put his instructions into practice. I began to live as mindfully as I could, noticing my panicky mind states and working to let them go. I remember the day that someone on Facebook mentioned having a panic attack and I had the passing thought, "Hmmm, I haven't had one of those for several years." Then it hit me—I hadn't had a panic attack for years!

At my meditation instructor's suggestion, I started doing yoga. It wasn't long before pains and tightness that I had attributed to my age eased and disappeared. I started cleaning up my eating patterns and other patterns of material and social media consumption. I can honestly say that meditation, *asana*, and *pranayama* saved me.

I got a YogaFit Level One teacher certification to help others overcome their discomfort as well. Now I have embarked on a 200-hour certification and am helping others ease their pain and tension, both mental and physical.

And, oh, by the way, you know how I said at one point I thought I would never be happy? Well, I was wrong!

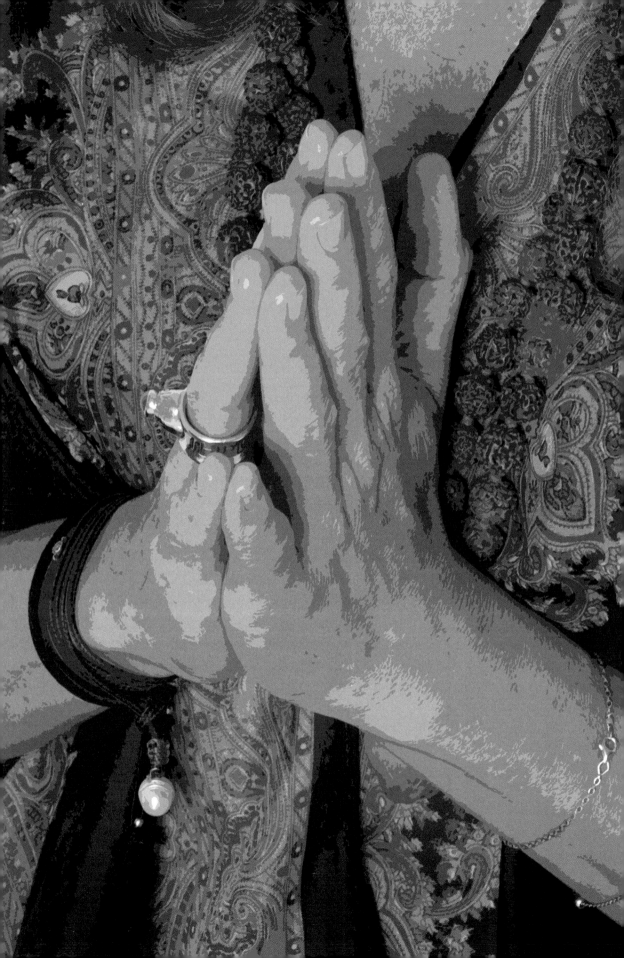

CHAPTER 3

How Yoga Heals Trauma

"One who is able to withdraw the senses from their objects, like a tortoise drawing its limbs within its shell, is firmly established in wisdom."

—BHAGAVAD GITA 2:58

I always say yoga teaches us to "get comfortable being uncomfortable." If yoga is new to you, using the mat as your "laboratory" is an excellent place to explore what it truly means to be uncomfortable. Facing your trauma and embracing the path to healing can feel uncomfortable, but showing up is a huge step. As mentioned in Chapter 2, the brain is rewired when trauma is experienced. Long term stress and trauma change the brain and body, and some of the changes may be permanent. The changes can in mood disorders and disease, addiction and self-esteem issues, anxiety and depression, lethargy and hopelessness, and destructive behavior. It is not uncommon for people to keep repeating this pain in their present-tense life by inviting in people and situations that will keep them in the trauma state. When you stop inviting the trauma in, you will have a sense of victory.

Studies are continuing to uncover the dramatic effects that various types of yoga and mindfulness have on brain function, mood, and disease mortality rates.

Healing comes from rebalancing and reversing the impact that trauma did to the brain. Through yoga and being able to breathe, flow, and self-talk our way through the most challenging yoga positions and holds, you are staying present and calming the nervous system. When we practice yoga, we get to simply "show up" for ourselves. You will hear me say throughout this book, "just show up for yourself." For those of us dealing with trauma symptoms, we already know what it's like to be uncomfortable, and ironically, in many situations, those with trauma feel comfortable in their trauma. Practicing yoga gives us the control to experience those places of physical and mental discomfort and not only get comfortable with them, but—even more poignant—learn to work with them and through them.

When it comes to healing, it is important to acknowledge the trauma, accept the trauma, and take action to become resilient. The good news is, humans are resilient. And in the case of trauma, rewiring the brain back to relaxation is possible if you show up.

Yoga teaches us to be in our bodies and minds as both the witness and participant. It simultaneously connects us to ourselves and shows that we are connected to a force much bigger than ourselves. Yoga unifies all aspects of self: dark and light, despair and joy, suffering and pleasure. We learn to accept all aspects of self, in a non-dualistic, dialectal way. The dualistic mind cannot process things like infinity, mystery, God, grace, suffering, sexuality, death, or love. Nondual consciousness is a holistic knowing, where your mind, heart, soul, and senses are open and receptive to the moment just as it is, which allows you to love things in themselves and as themselves, including yourself.

It can be said that yoga helps us accept whatever our trauma is and whatever situation caused it by helping to create this no-dualistic consciousness. If we can accept infinity, we can accept our trauma; acceptance is the second step after acknowledgement. Yoga helps us acknowledge (or in my case, allow for the memory to surface), accept, and take action for ourselves and for others. Yoga is action and creates a space for more action. For me, yoga has been the gateway that opened the door to deeper spiritual and psychological seeking, activities, and experiences. The process of yoga keeps opening doors and, by entering into those rooms, we find not only more doors, but ourselves in the process. Yoga helps you find and connect to yourself—what could be more healing than that? Returning to source energy, higher consciousness, and the infinite space of the Universe—that heals.

Buddha said that pain and suffering are part of the process of life and growth. You are not defined by your trauma, but trauma makes you part of who you are. Trauma is an experience response rooted in survival.

What ends up being traumatic to each person is unique and symptoms will vary depending on life circumstances, previous experiences, and other factors. Trauma and PTSD are garnering much attention in America in recent years, and there are many different types of treatment from cognitive and behavioral therapy to somatic or body therapy. Traditional cognitive and behavioral therapy, or the "top-down" approach as previously discussed, has not proven to be very effective for trauma victims and PTSD sufferers, and therapists are turning more toward somatic therapies or a "bottom-up" approach. Body-based or bottom-up treatments like yoga relieve symptoms of PTSD by resetting the nervous system. Yoga also helps trauma victims create a connection with their body that they have lost; in turn, they regain a sense of control, which is one of the critical goals in trauma treatment. Yoga also helps trauma survivors build internal strength through mindfulness and is gaining acceptance as trauma treatment and healing among the therapy community.

Scaer's *The Body Bears the Burden: Trauma, Dissociation, and Disease* also speaks to the essential ingredients of successful somatic treatment, all of which are addressed in yoga:

- **Rituals:** Repetitive movement with breath takes participants into a brainwave state known as alpha. In the alpha state, participants are more relaxed and open to the affirmative statements offered through YogaFit transformational language

- **Integration of Cerebral Hemispheres:** During arousal or stress, some portions of our left brain hemisphere are inhibited. It appears that the right amygdala, when operating singly, increases the arousal. When there is integration of both hemispheres, the amygdala goes offline. Eye movements (focus on object or *drishti*), counting (focus on counting breath), and singing (chanting), all may increase integration of the hemispheres.

- **Empowerment:** Several experts state that empowerment is the ultimate goal of all trauma therapy. Trauma victims feel helpless and overwhelmed by their circumstances and life. The Essence of YogaFit tells the participant that they are in charge. We ask our students to listen to their bodies and make decisions based on how they are feeling in the present moment, and we make it OK to modify every pose.

Recalling the Essence of YogaFit is important here—letting go of competition and expectation so that we don't cloud our mind with attachment. Success and failure are equally important on our journey, and neither require judgment.

In general, we want to focus on bottom-up processing with slower, more limbic-brain activated movements that help you find your inner healing mechanisms. The path forward is through the trauma, which the body and mind have been avoiding at all costs. The body and mind have, in fact, oriented themselves around the trauma so that you feel safe from ever having to go back to that place again. Those are the irrational behaviors, addictions, unhealthy relationship patterns, that function to protect your body.

Looking at it from a different perspective, that place is held sacred to some degree as sometimes a trauma survivor's entire life literally revolves around the trauma to include building bridges, roads, and shortcuts that function as detours around the crime scene. However, the path to healing is through the hole created—not around it. Once we start to pick up the pieces, bit-by-bit and feeling-by-feeling, we find our way back to the very place we have been avoiding. In doing so, we allow the body to release the trauma. That is why bottom-up processing is so effective. We start rebuilding at the somatic level, putting the pieces back together so that we have an integrated whole person when we are done in body, mind, and spirit. We believe that is the gift of trauma.

Bottom-up processing guidelines include:
- Reconnect to the bones first, especially the pelvis
- Focus on the psoas and psoas release poses (a sequence for this is in later chapters)
- Move slower—slower movement awakens the limbic or emotional brain

Specific Benefits of Yoga for Trauma

Parasympathetic Nervous System

Yoga activates the parasympathetic nervous system (PNS) and transitions us from our stuck state of "fight or flight" (SNS) back into "rest and digest" (PNS). When you stimulate the PNS, you're able to restore balance, and lower your heart rate and blood pressure. The PNS and the SNS are like a seesaw; when one goes up, the other one goes down. If your SNS is constantly in action, your cortisol goes up and your adrenals become depleted. By activating the PNS and lowering cortisol, you find balance.

Vagus Nerve Activation Helps Us Reactivate the PNS

The vagal pathway is a system of nerves that connects the brain to the body, and regulates many organs in the body—heart, lungs, gut, and liver. Your brain and nervous system tell your organs what to do and when your vagus nerve is impacted by your trauma, it may malfunction and not cooperate with your body as normal. Yoga reduces overall stress and yoga breathing and guided exercises increase vagal tone effectively, managing and activating the PNS.

Yoga Teaches You to Listen and Honor the Body

Through our yoga practice we develop a better relationship with our bodies including how we treat and speak to them. Yoga is body centered. Unlike the mind, the body doesn't lie. Yoga uses the simplicity of feeling the body and teaches our minds to listen to our bodies and honor them

Yoga Helps You Identify with Your Emotions

Yoga shows us how to become the witness, when we watch from a calm centered place we can more easily identify emotions.

Our Thoughts Create Feelings

Yoga is for the body and mind but through the body, yoga helps us identify emotions which are reactions to our thoughts. In some poses you may feel fear, joy, or grief because your body and your emotions are connected. If you hurt yourself in class, you will feel negative emotions. In some poses, you will have a surge of positive emotions. Almost any physical exercise floods the brain with chemicals to trigger responses. A mindful yoga practice helps us manage what the body is doing and how the mind and emotions are reacting to this information.

Yoga Helps Rewire Your Brain

The brain is deeply impacted by trauma. However, with proactive self-care, it can be reversed to a normal state and thus not allowing your trauma to take complete control of your life. Yoga, due to its calming affects to the central nervous system, can greatly aid (with continual practice) in the recovery and rebalance of the brain. Yoga releases gamma-aminobutyric (GABA), a calming agent produced by the brain. When the body is stressed, GABA levels are lowered and adrenaline is increased. It's important to the mind and body that GABA is regulated so that your nervous system is calm. Unfortunately, drugs and alcohol can stimulate the GABA and replicate the calming affects normally produced by GABA naturally. This is a reason why the reliance on substances is dangerous for the mind and body, because they trick you into the good feel that the natural body produces when it is taken care of.

If you do yoga regularly, it has been shown that GABA can maintain its regulatory levels. It is scientifically proven that yoga relieves stress. When your brain is not in ongoing stress, your body will learn to recalibrate and not rely on the stress the trauma has made it accustomed to.

Staying Present in the Moment

Showing up for yourself on your mat is important. Yoga requests that we remain alert while feeling our bodies in the poses. One of the best "stay present" techniques I use is what we teach in YogaFit's Level Two Communication Training—starting a positive running dialog with your body in the practice. I do this by noticing what I'm feeling in my body with each movement, like if my hamstrings are feeling tight or how does my shoulder feel today? Again without judgement or expectation, speak and observe the answer.

Survivor story: Laura

I am a veteran who has found the importance of the air we breathe.

I served fifteen years in the military with numerous deployments and a six-month tour to Afghanistan in 2006. It was not until several years later in 2015 that I was diagnosed with PTSD, anxiety, and depression, with a medical release in 2017. Having many bodily injuries, medical issues, uncertainty of where my life was going to go, as well as mental health issues, I was lost. Bricks weigh a lot; the more you add on, the heavier they get. This was how my chest felt. No matter what I could do or try to do, there was always something taking the air away from me. Many people would tell me, "You need to do yoga." Never did they say what kind, yet I still felt I could not. I could not because, besides the injuries, my mind would never stop going. Even when I would try to sleep at night, it felt like there was a freight train just going through so many thoughts on anything and everything—flashbacks, sounds. I could not handle that anymore, but I really did not want to be medicated.

As I was just scrolling through Facebook one day, I came upon an ad for YogaFit. "Hmm, let's check this out." I clicked the link and started going through what was available, and then it was there in front of me: YogaFit for Warriors Trauma-Sensitive Yoga. I read what it involved and thought, "Why not; what do I have to lose?

I attended the course and, well, I will tell you the first day—actually the first hour—was so emotional and difficult for me. Yet I was there for a reason; I was there for me. As the course progressed, I was given information by the trainer on how the brain works and how the body works. One word: Breath. From there, I learned how to belly breathe; nostril breathe; inhale for four, exhale for four. Now just because I was given these tools, it did not help me right away. I completed the course and headed back home.

The triggers were still there all around me: the weapons firing from the army base, the choppers flying overhead, the transport trucks driving down the highway; the list could go on. As the heaviness in my chest began, I would put one hand on my heart one hand on my stomach inhale, exhale, focus; again inhale, exhale, focus. As weeks went on, I learned within myself that this breathing was helping me, yet my mind was still racing. Going back into my books from the course and reviewing poses that we were taught for trauma, I started to practice. Some of the poses that gave me comfort (not in the beginning) were: Bound Angle, Easy Seated Pose, Upward Facing Dog, Downward Facing Dog, Warrior One, and Warrior Two; I am just starting to introduce headstands into my practice. These poses give me the chance to slow my body down with my breath, which, in turn, slows down my nervous system, allowing me to stay in parasympathetic. The adrenaline slows down, and I am able to breathe without the weight on my chest. My lungs fill up; I feed and nourish my body. Now, when I have triggers, and I still do, I breathe and look around for things I can see, touch, smell, and taste.

My spouse also did many deployments and a six-month tour to Afghanistan in 2005. He had several attempts on his life and turned to alcohol. He was not diagnosed with PTSD until around 2012. His body was failing him as he was drinking heavily, and suicidal thoughts were always there. He was at a point in life that giving up was much easier, or at least he thought that way. His career was also ending, and he was not able to get past anything. He stayed at home and drank. It was not until one day that he realized he was killing himself very slowly and painfully; in his own body, he was not able to breathe properly from weight gain and organs not working as a system.

He was released from the military and was given a chance for rehabilitation. This is a man who never really cared for physical activity or yoga. He was in rehab for three months, and during this time, he started to attend the different activities, and one that he truly liked was the yoga portion. He would tell me, "I am not really able to get into some on the postures yet, but we were shown how to deep breathe. My lungs expand so far, it's like being given a second chance at my life."

He began walking daily up to the point that he was walking over twenty kilometers every day. His weight started to drop, and he could breathe. He mentioned one day that he felt like he was walking on air because he was shown how to breathe, something we do every day, yet are we properly giving our body a chance to work as a team? He was given many tools while in rehab to help with his on-going triggers, and breathe one-two-three-four was one of them.

Like he said, no-one knows what you're doing except you. As you calm the body, you calm the mind, and that allows you to stay in the moment. He said to me one day, "I really never understood that fight, flight, freeze and the parasympathetic and sympathetic until I was in rehab."

We both now enjoy our days and are able to go out shopping and be in traffic because, when anxiety tries to overcome us, we breathe.

Without breath, there is no life. We accept that now and have incorporated yoga into our lives and into our community.

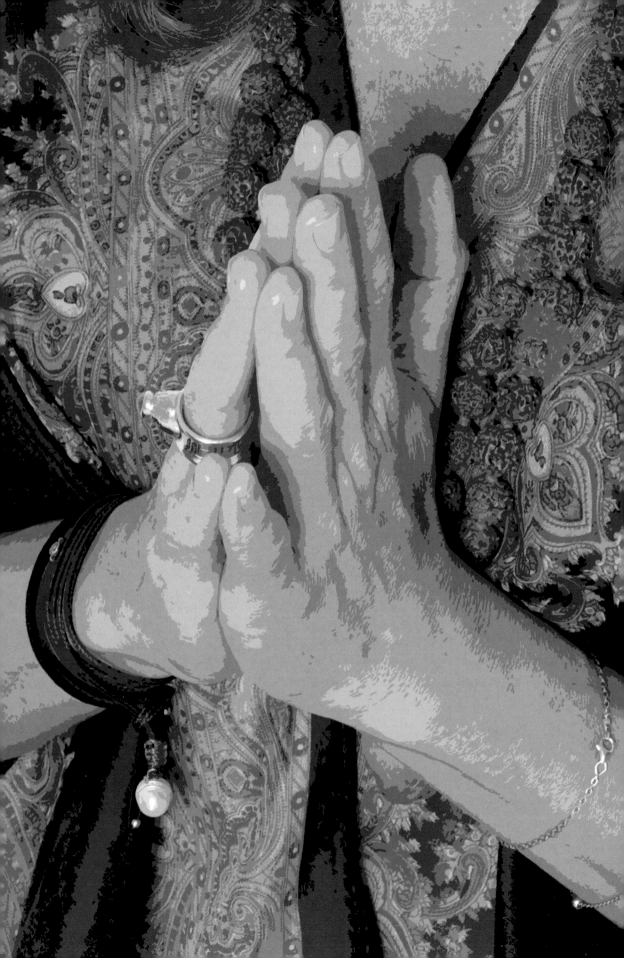

CHAPTER 4

Applications of Yoga: Breathing

"As a boat on the water is swept away by strong wind and thrown off course, even one of the senses on which the mind focuses can carry away one's intelligence."

—BHAGAVAD GITA 2:67

"As long as you're breathing and feeling, you're having a successful practice."

—BETH SHAW

"The mind is lord of the senses, but the breath is lord of the mind,"

—BKS IYENGAR

Pranayama, or breath as described in the Eight Limbs, has a profound effect on the body and mind. In YogaFit trainings, we say it simply, "Breath unites the body and mind." Breathing is the pathway to mindfulness, clarity and physical awareness.

Pranayama consists of two words, *Prana* and *Yama*. *Yama* is the same word used in the ethical rules of Patanjali's *Yoga Sutras* and they are the restraints. Prana is the energy of life and links with all the chemical processes in the body, from the burning of oxygen and glucose to every muscular contraction, glandular secretion, and thought. Learning to control your breath enhances energy, increases metabolism, and will allow you to feel, heal, and be present in the moment.

If we can control the breath, we can control the flow of *prana*, and according to the yoga tradition, if we can control the *prana*, we can control the subtle mechanics of our bodies, and alleviate the stresses trauma causes the nervous system.

Breathing is something we all do, but sometimes I feel like I forget to breath and actually wonder if I am even breathing. What I am really sharing here is that, like myself, you too may be a shallow breather and you may need to remind yourself, like I do, to breathe. Fortunately, the minute I start to practice yoga, my *ujjayi* breath (controlled, victorious breathing through the nose) kicks in, and as I'm dropping into meditation, I always increase my breath. When I work out, especially during swimming, I use a very focused breath. The beautiful thing about YogaFit is that we literally match breath with movement. This causes the mind and body to become one.

Our bodies innately breathe automatically without thought. There are however, many things that restrict and affect our breathing, momentarily and habitually. Slouching and bad posture collapse the lungs and restrict healthy pathways for the breath. Stress, pressure, and emotions create convulsive breathing patterns that trigger rapid heart rate and increased blood pressure. Muscle tension distresses the inhale and the exhale patterns.

People suffering from trauma symptoms often experience shortness of breath associated with panic attacks, and when the brain and vagus nerves are out of balance because of trauma, conscious and diaphragmatic breathing lowers the stress responses associated with "fight or flight." When we get scared or stressed, we sometimes hold our breath or lose control of it, and for many people dealing with the effects of trauma, shortness of breath can become a big problem. Studies have concluded that pranayama, or breath-control exercises, have great healing benefits for those with PTSD.

Our breath intimately affects our nervous system and is connected to our stress response. For example, when our breath is quick and shallow, it increases stress hormones, including cortisol and adrenalin. When it is controlled, it calms the body. Yoga practitioners have incorporated breathing practices for years because they understood the correlation between steady, controlled breath and mental and physical vitality. Modern science agrees that if your breath is out of control, fast, or shallow, it can cause many problems, including fatigue, sleep disorders, anxiety, heartburn, muscle cramps, dizziness, visual problems, chest pain, and heart palpitations. Learning how to breathe deeply both on and off the mat can reduce or even eliminate the majority of stress-induced symptoms.

When taking time to breathe with intention, we allow ourselves to be present in the moment, to slow down, and to evaluate impulse decisions. "Take ten deep breaths." According to the *Yoga Sutras, pranayama* practice also helps with the limbs of *dharana* (concentration), *dhyana* (meditation), and *Samadhi* (physical connection or oneness). Breath lies at the core of these limbs and not only fuels all of our bodily functions, but also helps with mental clarity and focus. Often, traumatized people feel nothing or feel rage (Levine, *Healing Trauma*, 2008), and this rage is expressed in inappropriate ways. I can relate to this; under the surface, in a little pocket, I have a lot of intergenerational anger that can rise to the surface quickly. This is why I am so grateful for yoga, meditation, and mindfulness.

There are as many ways to breathe as there are people. The basic guidelines in working with trauma-affected people—or anyone who is feeling out of balance mentally, emotionally, or physically—is to meet them where they are with the breath. If you are feeling anxious, start with an energizing breath and work towards a more relaxing breath. If you are feeling depressed or lethargic physically, start with a relaxing breath and work your way up to a balanced or more energizing breath. I love breath of fire, which is explained on the pages that follow. Bringing awareness to the breath creates a positive effect.

For the simple deep breathing exercises, the results are instantly noticeable and the practices are easy to learn on one's own. When starting with more complicated *pranayama* practices, it's helpful to have a teacher or video to watch.

Breath supplies our organs with oxygen. Oxygen purifies the blood stream and aides in the proper functioning of the brain, nerves, glands, and other internal organs. It also gives your organs the energy and rejuvenation they need to thrive. If your body is starved for oxygen, your blood is affected, and that hunger for oxygen causes quick and shallow breathing. When we practice yoga, we tap into this vital nutrient and center ourselves with a sound flow of breath from one pose to the next. I'm always trying to take those breathing patterns off the mat.

Mentally, steady breath will positively affect your well-being because it cleanses, focuses and relaxes the mind. If your breathing fluctuates in any way, whether through shortness or quickness of breath, it will trigger your psyche to react. When you take a moment to slow your breath, your respiratory system is calmed, as is your heart rate.

How do you tap into the breath?

Let's begin with the nose. In yoga, we use "nose-breathing only." Breathing through the nose instead of the mouth gives a sense of control and also is a natural defense mechanism to ward off germs. The nose also leads to a passageway line with mucus membranes that warms cold air and catches outside elements.

Breath patterns have an important link to our nervous systems. Our breath is the gateway to activate our parasympathetic nervous system (PNS). The PNS is the "rest and digest" mode, our calming, healing nervous system. Shallow chest breathing activates our sympathetic nervous system (SNS) and creates higher heart rates and more overall tension. Slow deep breathing does the opposite and is proven by peer-reviewed western science–published studies to be linked to better heath.

While there are many levels of *pranayama* practice, the more advanced practices would benefit from a teacher.

Dirga Pranayama (three-part breathing) is a simple and effective *pranayama* that all people can practice with no contraindications. The three parts are belly, ribs, and upper chest. It's great for insomnia, relieving stress and anxiety and to begin to breath more fully thus increasing the oxygen. The easiest way to practice is lying on your back with one hand on the chest and the other on the belly. It can also be practiced in a chair. Breathe in and feel your breath fill up the belly, then the chest, and the last sip of air, lifts the clavicle. Then exhale top to bottom, upper chest, rip cage, and belly.

Equal Parts Breathing is another beginner *pranayama* practice. Start by lying down and become aware of the natural rhythm of your breath. Inhale for a count of four and then exhale for a count of four. It should be a count that is easy to accomplish. If you find yourself holding your breath or the breath getting difficult, try an easier count.

Nadi Shodhana Pranayama (alternate nostril breathing) is one of the most common pranayama practices and is therapeutic for most everyone. This breath balances both sides of your body, the right and left brain, the creative and analytical, and our male and female energy. It calms and centers the body and mind. It is not recommended that people with heart disease, high blood pressure, or ulcers pass the beginner level.

1. Do a simple breath-focus exercise to start (close your eyes and take ten deep breaths, focusing on how your body feels and scanning your body for any pain, injury, or special conditions, as well as parts of your body that feel energized), then raise your right hand to your face with your palm facing in.

2. Take your right hand and, with your fingers outstretched, block off your right nostril by putting gentle pressure on it with your thumb. Be sure to keep the rest of your fingers straight and pointing up toward the sky. Your fingers act like antennas for more energy.

3. With a long, slow, deep breath, gently inhale through your left nostril. Then release your thumb and, using the index finger of your right hand, block off your left nostril and exhale long, slowly, and completely, through your right nostril.

4. Keeping your left nostril blocked with your index finger, inhale slowly and fully through your right nostril.

5. Switch your fingers again so that your right thumb is blocking your right nostril and exhale completely through your left nostril.

6. Continue to alternate with one complete inhale and exhale per thumb or finger.

Ujjayi Pranayama (victorious breath) can be practiced in any position and occurs naturally in deep sleep. It creates heat and one-point focus and cleanses one's nervous system. It is achieved by constricting the vocal chords and sounds like a scuba tank or a loud growling whisper. Not to be practiced by people with heart disease. Those with low blood pressure should correct it first before practicing this pranayama.[8] It is also not recommended for pregnant woman because it is heating.

Breath of Fire (*Kapalabhati*) uses deep, rapid breath cycles to warm your body and increase your energy. Traditionally, the Breath of Fire is not

---

8   ibid pg193

a pranayama technique but rather a *kriya*, or cleansing practice. Many of the toxins in your body are released during your exhale, which is the focus here. Practice it during Mountains I and III. Some of the effects: it energizes and activates the right side of your pranic system, stimulates your nervous system, and cleanses your respiratory system.

Practice:

1. Find a comfortable seated or reclining position
2. Begin inhaling through your nose, keeping your mouth closed.
3. Exhale half the air out of your lungs to a point somewhere between exhale and inhale.
4. Your exhale should be quick and sharp, contracting your abdominal muscles. In this exercise, exhalations are short, vigorous, and active; inhalations are light and passive.
5. Continue this rhythmic pattern for twenty to twenty-five breaths. Repeat two to five rounds, finishing with a deep Three-Part Breath.

Simhasana Pranayama (lion's breath) relieves tension, helps ease the mind, and stimulates the immune system. To practice lion's breath, sit on your heels with your hands resting on your knees, take a deep breath in, and when you exhale, open your mouth, stick out your tongue and make a loud "Haaaa" as you exhale all the breath. The breath should pass the back of the throat. Bad knees? Sit in a chair.

Even just sitting where you are a taking deep, calming breaths has an instant effect on one's body and mind. Because these practices can be very strong, it is always recommended to employ safe breathing practices.

- Consult your physician prior to doing advanced breathing techniques or breath-suspension.
- Learn your favorite breathing practice and do it outside in the morning when the air is fresh.
- Wear loose, non-restrictive clothing.
- Avoid areas with polluted air, including rooms with smoke from candles and incense.
- If you are sick or have asthma, lung issues, or heart disease, refrain.
- If you are pregnant, avoid breath of fire and breath-suspension.
- Avoid suspending your breath if you have high blood pressure—it can temporarily raise your blood pressure.

- Stop if you feel dizzy or lightheaded.
- Remain relaxed throughout the entire breath exercise.

Those with asthma, lung issues (COPD, emphysema, chronic bronchitis, etc.), and heart disease (hypertension, congestive heart failure, cardiovascular disease) may want to be extra cautious or avoid this all together.

If you are still having challenges, consider going to a respiratory therapist for breath retraining to learn ways to engage effective breath. You can actually learn to utilize the diaphragm and accessory muscles more effectively, improve lung function, and lower blood pressure. YogaFit trainer Patti Bain is a respiratory therapist and helped craft this chapter.

Once we stop breathing, we cease to exist in the human form, so breathe big and breathe bold!

Survivor story: Lisa

My love for yoga started over ten years ago when I began taking classes taught by an inspiring, gifted, and giving teacher. I fell in love with her fast-moving yoga classes, and occasionally opted for her slower, gentler hatha classes. In late 2013, my husband (second marriage) was killed in a tragic motorcycle crash. We had been together eight years. My kids, who at the time were ages fifteen and eighteen, were devastated as they loved him very much. Within days after the funeral, I was told by his sister, my sister-in-law, that he had been having an affair with one of my best friends. In the months following, I learned that he lived a double life, having many affairs. After his death, I felt like I was grieving two losses—his life and the loss of what I thought was reality, our marriage. In early 2014, I decided to retire early from my longstanding career in federal law enforcement. I wasn't functioning at my best and knew I had to leave a career that I loved. Immersing myself in yoga classes, I would find myself crying and my body shaking uncontrollably. This happened a lot. My teacher always sensed when it would start, and she would work us into a pose so others wouldn't have a clear shot of me as we were facing mirrors. I'd glance at her face and see her concern, her tears. When this first started to happen, it scared me. But as it continued, I began to not care and feel ashamed. I noticed how I felt drastically better after class, in body, mind, and soul. Sometimes I would get so lost in my thoughts that I'd have no memory of the entire class. Other times, my mind brought me to places it hurt me to be, but then I'd shake and tremble and feel better when it was over. I'd find myself in deep connection with God, almost as if he was standing there holding my hand. Yoga became the place I could go and experience healing of my body, mind, and soul.

I decided to take a leap and start YogaFit training. Whether I taught or not, I wanted to learn the basics in case I decided to teach. In early 2015, I completed Level 1. It was a wonderful experience and I knew I wanted to continue. Then my life changed once more. In March 2015, I found my son unconscious on a Sunday morning, barely breathing. Long story short, he overdosed and was in a coma. His kidneys and liver had shut down, and he had brain damage. Within the first week of him being in Intensive Care, the doctors told me I would need to make a decision to place him in a facility or pull all life support. I told him he was nuts and that it was way too soon to have such a discussion. My son was going to make it. With the power of love and prayer, he walked out of the hospital in a month's time, fully recovered. Or was he? In the following months, my son shared with me about his drug use, and that his step-dad not only knew about it, he also used with my son and his friends. I wanted him to get counseling after everything that happened, and he refused, saying there was no point talking to a stranger about the past. He wanted to move forward, doing all the right things to stay healthy. Life proceeded in a positive direction the next year or so, then my life changed forever. On July 3, 2016, a mother's worst nightmare occurred, as my son died in his sleep on the couch at a friend's house from an overdose of a prescription medication, oxycodone.

The tragedy and trauma of his passing will be felt in my entire being for the rest of my life, and in the lives of my daughter, and my ex-husband. The stigma of addiction is ugly, and its effects on the family, devastating. There is so much guilt, shame, blame, anger, helplessness, hopelessness, and sadness. Living through grief and the "new normal," you realize you can't go back to who you used to be or what you used to do. I remember seeing a Facebook post by YogaFit about a yoga training to help those with PTSD. I read about it, and wondered if I had PTSD. I believed I did, and wanted to take the YogaFit for Warriors training. Although I wanted to help myself by learning about trauma and yoga for warriors, I was considering using it to help others suffering from addiction. What I learned during the training came full circle. My body's reaction of crying, shaking, and trembling during earlier yoga classes, where the trainer used deep, slow, and gentle poses, was actually bringing healing by releasing the trauma that hijacked my entire being.

The process of healing has taken me to places that I could have never imagined myself going. It was that "new normal" again, stepping out of my comfort zone to channel my pain and grief into helping myself first, then others. I also wanted to learn everything there is to know about the disease of addiction, things I should've known but didn't. So I went back to college to study mental health and addiction with the goal of becoming a Licensed Chemical Dependency Counselor, which I'm still in the process of. I've had the pleasure of completing an internship, working at a treatment center to help those afflicted with drug and alcohol disorders. I stepped out of my comfort zone and led a yoga class for the group I was working with at the treatment center. Treatment centers everywhere want to offer yoga as part of recovery because of its mind-body-spiritual connections and healing, but many haven't figured out how to do that. The treatment center I interned at let me do one class. Set to calming music, a song called "Angels Voices," I led them into a series of very gentle and slow basic poses. I'll never forget the joy I felt watching them let themselves go and focus only on what they were doing in the present moment. Afterwards, I witnessed the calmness in their faces and movements. I heard them talk about how much better they felt, and they loved the soothing music. One young man told me before class that there was no way he could do yoga. I just told him to do whatever he could. Afterwards, he came up to me saying that he really liked it and he hadn't felt that good or had this much energy in a long time. From that experience, I realized the value of yoga in treating the trauma of addiction, and why it's essential in recovery.

Stepping out of my comfort zone again, I agreed to temporarily offer free yoga classes to the kids at a Juvenile Detention Center. Not knowing anything about these kids, yet knowing they suffered some type of trauma that led them there, the first ten minutes or so—and for some the entire first class—was tense. Eventually, they were willing to let go of their tough exteriors and reluctance to participate. They learned how they can control and use their breath and movement to rid themselves of negative thoughts and feelings. Most importantly, they learned how to feel respected and valued, and that they have the power to control their outcome in a positive, healthy way.

I'm so very grateful how God placed my first yoga teacher into my life, giving her the gift of yoga to share with others, which she does so compassionately and with love, which has saved me during the darkest moments of my life. He continues to lead me down new paths that involve helping others who suffer. I continue to take one day at a time, choosing to live in the present moment where I feel safe and loved. Whether I continue as a yoga student only, or develop my practice and instruction into using yoga as a means for healing addiction and mental health disorders or any other source of trauma, I know that it will bring continued healing and hope.

CHAPTER 5

Applications of Yoga: Physical Practice

"Be steadfast in yoga, O Arjuna. Perform your duty without attachment, remaining equal to success or failure. Such equanimity of mind is called yoga."

—BHAGAVAD GITA 2:48

"Nothing gets between me and my mat."

This mantra came to me almost a decade ago when a relationship I was in went from an almost-marriage to a devastating break up within days. February 15, one day after Valentine's Day, it was over. I was a walking zombie, in so much pain, and of course I had to go to a YogaFit conference where I knew no one wanted to see me in a down place. Part of my work, I believe is to lift people's spirits and I can never let my emotions or challenges get in the way of that. Going to that "Mind-Body Fitness" conference in Virginia, miles away from where I was supposed to get married, was truly a blessing. Part of any recovery is to be of service and nothing pulls me out of my "stuff" faster than having to show up for others. While teaching the master class, the phrase "nothing comes between me and my mat" came to me. I liked it so much, I created an advertising campaign using that mantra. Many days when I just don't feel like practicing, I will schedule a class so that I am forced to just show up for myself.

Showing up for yourself is both powerful and empowering. Allow yourself to make your yoga practice an inquiry into self. When I get into a dark room, and get into my body, I often just witness the physical: "my hips are tight today," "that headstand feels good," "my balance is off." The more we can observe the physical, the more we train ourselves to observe our thoughts and emotions. Observing the physical can also be very meditative.

The beauty of yoga is its flexibility. Our yoga practice will always hold space for us and meet us where we need to be met. Though some days we may need a more uplifting practice and other days something more calming. The following sequences are designed to meet your needs as they arise. When dealing with trauma, anxiety, PTSD, and depression, every day is as unique as the weather. I know I have days when I just want to cry on my mat and days when I want to push my practice to the limits with extra pushups and a lot of heat. My best advice is to let your body guide you as feelings and emotions can be a lot more transient than how your body feels in a particular day. It's all about just making it to your mat.

A daily yoga practice combined with journaling can help identify patterns and can be used as a self-diagnostic tool. There are days when it will be difficult to practice. Those days, just sit on your mat and breathe. A key component is staying in the right headspace is the creation of daily rituals. Allow your practice to be a strong part of that foundation. Remember, conscious awareness of our thoughts, feelings, actions, reactions, and behaviors is a muscle we need to strengthen daily.

YogaFit Seven Principles of Alignment

In YogaFit, we express hatha yoga postures using our Seven Principles of Alignment (SPA). These principles help to create the optimal biomechanical position for the body during movement and while holding the poses. SPA increases safety while simultaneously providing functional mechanical principles that you can use in your daily life. YogaFit SPA helps us practice, understand, and self-correct and the Essence of YogaFit helps us accept ourselves and protects us when we are dealing with trauma—our own or others. Safety is paramount, especially for those wounded emotionally, spiritually, mentally, and psychologically.

Here are the Seven Principles of Alignment:

1. **Establishing Base and Dynamic Tension:** Establish a firm base in the feet and hands, stacking your joints for maximum support and contracting your muscles to become stable in a pose.

2. **Creating Core Stability:** Use the muscles of the trunk (for instance, the abdominals and the erector spinae) to create core stability prior to moving into and while holding poses for greater strength and internal support.

3. **Aligning the Spine:** The spine is supported through core stabilization in all applicable poses, and the head follows the movement of the spine. When moving into twists, flexion, or extension, start in neutral spine.

4. **Softening and Aligning Knees:** In all applicable poses, the knees stay in line with the ankles and point directly out over the toes. In general, the knees, when bent, will also remain in the same line as the hips. To prevent hyperextension, keep a micro-bend in the knees at all times.

5. **Relaxing Shoulders Back and Down:** The shoulders are drawn naturally back and down in poses to help reduce tension in the neck and shoulders.

6. **Hinging at the Hips:** When moving into and out of forward bends, hinge from the hips, using the natural pulley system of the ball and socket joint and keeping a micro-bend in the knees.

7. **Shortening the Lever:** When hip-hinging, flexing, or extending the spine, keep the arms out to the side or alongside the body to reduce strain on the muscles of the lower back.

Inner Dialogue

Without a positive inner dialogue, you're not going to get very far. Self-talk can make or break us. In YogaFit we practice giving PEP (Praise-Encourage-Praise) feedback to others, and I want you to learn to apply this feedback when communicating with yourself during times of struggle.

In groups, to help each other improve, PEP feedback is a great way for you to shift your dialogue to carefully support those around you. This format is also used to guide you through self-talk and build a safer inner dialogue when you feel frustrated or need to talk yourself out of something.

Start with a positive statement, then encourage with a strong help statement, followed by another positive statement. Below are the PEP guidelines when speaking to others. Learning this will help us communicate better in our relationships. Once you gain an understanding of PEP, you can use it on yourself. I use self-talk constantly.

Praise-Encourage-Praise

Principles of Giving Constructive Feedback

- With an intention of being helpful, supportive, and encouraging, ask permission before providing feedback.
- Focus first on the positive and then on how to improve. Deal only with a specific skill or technique that can be changed.
- Describe the skill or technique rather than evaluating it.
- Relate objectively what specifically was seen or heard. Facts about skill or technique are exact and without exaggeration.
- Use "I" statements to accept responsibility for your own perceptions and emotions.
- Check to make sure that the recipient understood the message in the way it was intended. Avoid making the recipient "wrong" by wanting to be "right."
- Avoid extreme or coercive language like "should," "always," and "never."

Principles of Receiving Feedback

- Listen openly and without excuses or judgments of yourself or others.
- When you ask for feedback, be specific in describing the skill or technique about which you want the feedback.

- Let go of defensive reactions or temptations to rationalize the skill or technique at issue.
- Summarize your understanding of the feedback.
- Using "I" statements, share your thoughts and feelings about the feedback.

Your inner coach should be your best advocate and always help you achieve your goals.

Three Mountain Format

Three Mountain Format, which is warm up, work, and cool down, has suggested modifications and options on most poses. During your pose sequences, I encourage you to apply the essence of YogaFit to be easy on yourself—listening to your body; letting go of judgment, expectation, and competition; and being present in the moment and in your practice. Use YogaFit SPA to keep your body safe.

In YogaFit, we apply modern exercise science to the ancient mind-body practice of yoga. While yoga can have a profound impact on the physical, emotional, and spiritual health of students, improper sequencing and pacing create opportunities for physical discomfort and injury. For this reason, I ask you to use the following format to establish full readiness and benefits from your poses.

Mountain 1: Warmup phase

Mountain 2: Work phase

Mountain 3: Cool-down phase

In addition to these three phases, I ask you to use two "valleys," which are extensions of Mountain 1 and Mountain 2, respectively:

Valley 1: Sun salutations

Valley 2: Upright standing balance poses

Importance of Warmup and Cool Down

Warming up the body completely with large body moves prior to engaging in any complex or flexibility-oriented pose is important to prep the muscles, especially if your workout environment is cold. Many assume that stretching prior to exercise or an athletic event helps to prepare the muscles for the activity and reduce injury. However, the scientific literature has not, to date, confirmed that flexibility exercises performed before the elevation of core body temperature are effective in reducing injury. Since yoga is a form of exercise that requires a combination of flexibility, strength, endurance, and coordination, I want you to stretch at the end.

The human body is composed of a number of structures: skeletal, muscular, nervous, circulatory, and so on. The muscular structure of the body provides movement and protection for the skeletal system. All actions in the body take place through the contraction or relaxation of muscles at the major joints. Each of these joints has an inherent range of motion due to the configuration of the bones in the body. However, this range of motion can be restricted by the ability of the soft tissues of the body, including the muscles, tendons (which attach muscle to bones), and ligaments (which connect bones together), to accommodate the range. Muscles can be become tense due to many factors, including stress and working joints through a restricted range of motion. The result is perceived inflexibility.

The solution to increasing flexibility is to begin working the joints through the full range of motion, which "stretches" the muscles and, to a lesser degree, the tendons. Two essential properties of muscles allow them to stretch: elasticity and plasticity. The elastic properties of muscles allow them to return back to their original state from a stretch. If this were not the case, muscles would lengthen continuously until they had become so loose that no movement was possible! The plastic properties of muscles allow them to adapt to the continued stresses that we place on them and retain these adaptations. If muscles were not plastic, then we would not be able to strengthen or stretch them; they would just stay the same after each activity. Interestingly, both of these qualities become more evident when there is an elevation in core body temperature. Another way of saying this is that muscles respond better if we work them when they are warm.

Therefore, the most appropriate place to introduce deep stretching (and even strength and endurance work) is after an elevation in body temperature sufficient to increase the potential for elasticity and plasticity in our muscles. Consequently, all physical exercise, including yoga, should begin with warmups that elevate core body temperature and use the full range of motion in the major joints. Once we have sufficiently elevated the core body temperature, we can then begin using movements that condition the body for greater strength, stretch, and flexibility. Our deepest flexibility stretches should occur near the end of class, when the body is warmest and elasticity and plasticity in the muscles are optimal.

Before applying this to your yoga practice, know that fitness moves are incorporated, such as sit-ups, push-ups, lunges, and holds. Transitions are smooth from pose to pose with the focus on a full-body workout; all body parts are worked equally. Modifications and levels are offered to suit the needs of several different students at different levels in the room. Encourage yourself to take breaks; let go of expectations, judgment, and competition; and do not push yourself past your limits—you will know when you've reached your limit if you listen and feel the signs your body is giving you.

The following are a series of sequences to help with serenity, calmness, and living in the now. Please note that for those with trauma related to physical violence such as kidnapping, rape, or domestic abuse, certain props can be very triggering—eye masks, straps and ties. Avoid using these in class or on your own. I also personally prefer softer props like blankets and bolsters instead of hard blocks. We want our restorative poses and practice to be soft and yielding. Please be mindful of this.

Warmup Sequence

- Flight of the Bird (five to seven minutes, one breath for each movement)
- Chair Flow (five times)
- Sun Salutations
- Flow Series
- Cat and Cow (ten to fifteen times, one breath for each movement)

Cool Down Sequence

- Spinal Twist
- Lying Down Spinal Twist
- Bridge
- Upside Down Pigeon

- Reclining Butterfly
- Dead Bug

Yoga for Anxiety versus Yoga for Depression

Many people who are diagnosed with depression, also suffer and are diagnosed with anxiety. While depression and anxiety are different, symptoms and feelings often feel the same. Try to remember that depression is linked to events that occur in the past. Anxiety is the fear of what may happen in the future. Differentiating between the two can help you understand how to alleviate the symptoms and work through it.

With yoga as a tool, those with anxiety need to focus on calming down while those with depression need to be uplifted. For both conditions, yoga aids in keeping you in the present, rather than the worries and feelings of the past or future.

Anxiety Symptoms Include:

- Excessive worry
- Restlessness
- Being easily fatigued
- Trouble concentrating
- Irritability
- Sleep disturbance
- Muscle tension

Poses for Anxiety

- Seated Forward folds
- Cat and Cow
- Knees to chest Restorative supported bridge pose
- Inversions such as shoulder stand or supported headstand—instantly get grounded.

Depression

Because depression deflates energy and mood, yoga poses that promote increased energy and blood flow are important, including opening up the body to release tension and allowing your mood to lift and endorphins to increase.

Depression symptoms include:

- Depressed mood
- Lack of interest in enjoyable activities
- Increase or decrease in appetite
- Insomnia or hypersomnia
- Slowing of movement
- Lack of energy
- Feelings of guilt or worthlessness
- Trouble concentrating
- Suicidal thoughts or behaviors

Mood Reset Sequence

- Sun salutations
- Back bends
- Camel pose
- Chest Expansion
- Bow Pose—From lying down

Mood-Lifting Sequence

- Sun Salutation
- Sunflowers
- Flight of the Bird
- Warrior One
- Warrior Two
- The Flow Series
- Triangle Pose

Calming Down—Restorative Yoga

These poses will reset your nervous system, taking you from the state of fight-or-flight, to rest. There are days that I feel tired, drained, and heavy with emotional paralysis. I use this sequence to relax or sometimes to "jump start" more movement to follow. I find that a little movement often leads to more movement, but you just need to get moving.

- Cat and Cow to warm up
- Seated Forward Fold
- Seated Spinal Twist
- Knees to chest
- Upside Down Pigeon
- Lying down spinal twist
- Dead Bug
- Supported bridge
- Reclining Butterfly
- Final Relaxation
- Legs Up Against Wall

Centering Workout

The core is the center of the body, holding it together to help you stand upright, move gracefully, and function. Strengthening your core will uplift your mood and create a stronger you. Remember your third chakra, your power center, is located in your core center. We want to enhance our personal power by focusing on this key mind-body center.

- Core Work
- Bridge lifts
- Cat and Cow
- Spinal balance
- Plank
- Side Plank
- Down Dog
- Crocodile

- Up dog or cobra
- Childs pose

Restorative Trauma Sequence

- Windshield Wipers
- Side lying relaxation
- Supported child's pose
- Supported prone or belly
- Supported Fish
- Supported corpse or *savasana*

Psoas Release

The psoas and the energetic muscles that are intimately connected with the psoas—like the iliacus in the pelvic floor and the diaphragm that regulates our breathing and ultimately the cardiovascular system—are unlike any "muscles" in the traditional sense in the body. Their energy is the primary response mechanism involved in the initial fight-or-flight response in the body. They very quickly and intelligently shunt energy from the rest and digest processes in the torso to our limbs to help us mobilize for our defense along the fight-flight-freeze spectrum of potential postures. This energetic sympathetic response happens in cases of physical or emotional trauma and after an intense life-threatening event and can result in a high allostatic load (the wear-and-tear) in the body. The psoas release sequence can help to intentionally release this high allostatic load and, in essence, push the reset button of the nervous system. This is especially important after traumatic events where the person was immobilized in fear or wasn't able to complete the process of defending themselves for whatever reason.

As mentioned earlier, we often see this release in animals after a traumatic event and it resembles shaking or erratic, seemingly uncontrollable, movements. This is natural in animals and humans, but we don't encourage or even embrace the idea of being physically like animals at the nervous-system level. Our society and western medicine doesn't acknowledge the need for or even allow the shaking that humans would do naturally if allowed to reduce the high allostatic load. An example of this in humans is after surgery or birth, oftentimes people will report uncontrollable shaking. Here is a psoas release sequence to help ease the tension:

- Start lying on your back with knees bent and feet flat—hands on belly to encourage relaxed belly-breathing. Stay here five minutes, focusing on gently lengthening the exhale.
- Hug one knee in and extend the other leg straight out of the hip along floor, allowing it to hover a couple of inches off the floor, then slowly start to lift and lower the extended leg no higher than one to two inches about ten times.
- Staying on the same extended leg, flex the foot, then rotate the entire inner leg open to the ceiling so the toes are pointed to the side. Slowly slide the leg out to the side a few inches then back in and rotate the leg back so the toes are pointing straight up to the ceiling. Repeat the sequence three to five times on the same leg.
- Staying on the same extended leg, place the heel gently on the ground. Slowly drag it in towards the body, bending the knee, and then push it back out multiple times.
- Switch legs and repeat entire sequence starting with hugging one knee in and extending the other leg.
- Flowing bridge (five times) slowly with a yoga block wedged between the thighs—squeeze and slightly internally rotate adductors, pushing block gently towards the ground without squeezing glutes, if possible.
- Knees to chest and rock gently side to side for a few minutes, noticing any changes or sensations in the hips or belly.
- Stay laying on your back and bring your knees directly over hips with shins parallel to ground and feet flexed. Place a block between your thighs then flow side to side slowly with arms out like a T, shoulders back and down. Bring knees slowly to one side, keeping them parallel while squeezing the block, only going as far as knees and feet can stay parallel and both shoulders can stay relaxed and down on the ground
- Reclined butterfly with palms of hands placed gently on tops of thighs while alternating pressing thighs away from hips and encouraging hip flexors to relax.

- Lift hips only a couple of inches off the mat without squeezing glutes or outer thighs. Hold for two minutes and focus on relaxed belly-breathing, noticing any tension patterns in shoulders and jaws and releasing it.

- After two minutes, set hips back down in reclined butterfly pose and start to slowly close legs together like a Venus fly trap a couple of inches and hold for two minutes, feeling the energetic connection and resistance between the thighs. Notice any shaking or trembling in in the legs, hips, or belly and let it happen.

- Repeat closing the legs two more times, a couple of inches closer each time, without releasing effort.

- After the third round, set feet flat on floor and notice and allow any trembling to flow through legs and feet to the ground for five minutes.

- Turn to side in fetal posture and gently observe any sensations, feelings, or memories that arise for five minutes.

- Option to turn to back or on belly for final resting pose for as long as needed.

Pose Breakdowns and Descriptions

MOUNTAIN

Benefit of the pose: Mountain Pose is a foundational pose. It is used often to begin practice and as a transition to other poses. Mountain is also your posture pose and a way for you to heighten your mind-body awareness. Having good posture and a strong mind-body connection will help you be alert and make your movements strong and efficient. It serves as a strong focal posture to begin a standing practice or to warm up with.

● **Getting into the Pose:** Stand with your feet at the top of your mat and observe your breath. From a strong connection to your mat, lift up through the arches of your feet. Activate your inner thighs and your pelvic floor and draw your belly in. Lengthen your spine and soften your shoulders back and down from your ears. Open your chest and shoulders so that your palms are facing out and bring your chin in slightly.

● **Holding the Pose:** Create dynamic tension throughout your body, awakening all your muscles. Breathe more deeply with every breath—into your belly, your rib cage, and then your chest. Feel your body and notice your mind. With each breath, become more aware and more present.

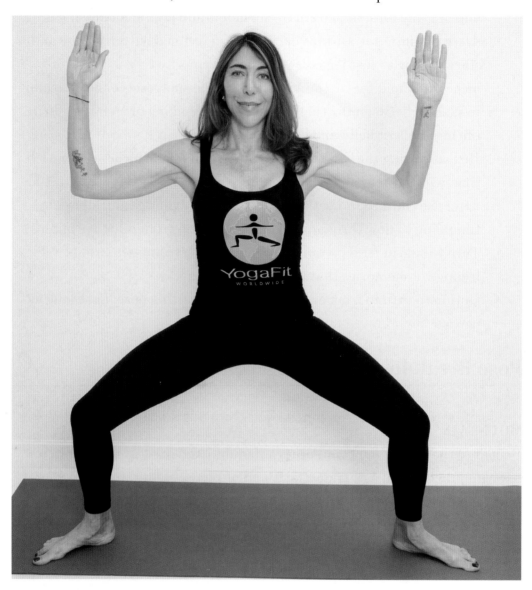

MOONFLOWER

● **Benefit of the pose:** Moonflowers build energy by working large muscle groups. Moonflowers work the legs and move the joints through a comfortable range of motion, while opening the chest. Benefits include strengthening of glutes, quads, hamstrings, abdominals, and shoulders.

● **Getting into the pose**: From Mountain Pose, step back to face the long edge of your mat, preparing for Moonflower. Open your thighs and turn your toes out. Inhale while raising your arms up and out for a five-pointed star and exhale into a squat. Your knees should track your toes, and your elbows should come into your ribs. Inhale, straighten your legs, reach your arms out; and exhaling, back into a squat. Move with your breath in Moonflowers.

● **Moving with the Pose:** Warm up your hips and shoulders in a comfortable range of motion.

SUNFLOWER

● **Benefit of the pose:** Sunflowers build energy by working large muscle groups and creating more pranic flow through the body. Sunflowers work the legs and move the joints through a comfortable range of motion. Benefits include strengthening of glutes, quads, hamstrings, abdominals, and shoulders.

● **Getting into the Pose:** Step back to face the long edge of your mat. Open your thighs and turn your toes out and your heels in for a plié squat. Inhale, bring arms overhead; exhale, and hinge forward from the hips, reaching your tailbone back. Keep a neutral spine as you sweep your arms toward the floor. Inhale back to starting position.

● **Moving with the Pose:** Continue to move through a comfortable range of motion as your body warms up. Step back to the top of your mat to continue your warmup.

● **Modifications:** If you have knee issues, limit your range of motion and stay in a comfortable place in the squat, pointing the knees over the center of the feet. For less intensity or shoulder concerns, place hands on thighs.

CHAIR

● **Benefit of the pose:** Chair Flow is a great workout for the lower body. It creates a lot of heat quickly as it works the largest muscle groups in the body. Chair Flow strengthens quads, glutes, shoulders, and core. To flow, move in and out of Chair Flow with every breath to warm up.

● **Getting into the Pose:** Bend your knees and drop your buttocks, as if you were sitting in a chair.

● **Holding the Pose:** Reach back with your tailbone. Lift your chest to the sky. Lift your arms parallel to the floor, keeping your elbows slightly bent. Support your lower back by engaging your core. Keep your knees behind your toes by shifting your weight to your heels.

● **Modifications:** Rest your hands on your thighs for more support.

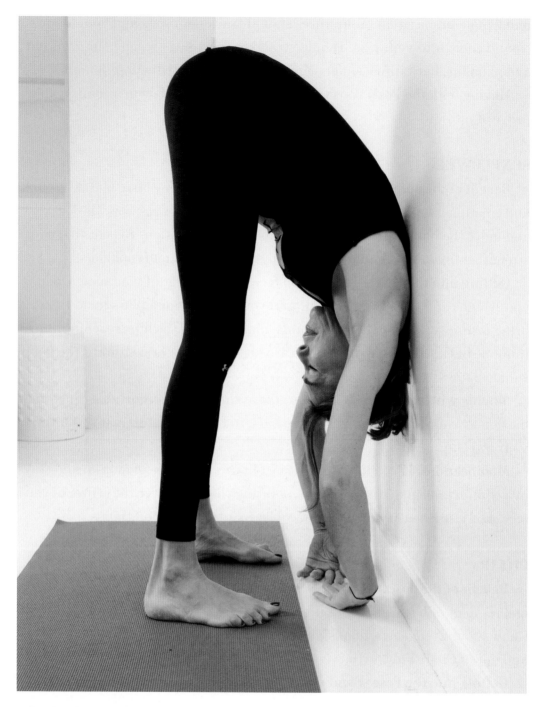

FORWARD FOLD

● **Getting into the Pose:** Start at the front of your mat in Mountain Pose. Inhale, sweeping your arms up; exhale, swan diving with your arms out to your sides and your knees bent. Bringing your hands to the floor or your shins. Option to straighten your legs for Forward Fold.

● **Holding the Pose:** In Forward Fold, allowing your head and neck to relax, shaking your head "no," nodding "yes."

● **Modifications:** Rest your hands on your thighs for more support

CHEST EXPANSION

● **Getting into the Pose:** From Mountain Pose, reach your palms toward one another behind your body. Stay here working on building strength or interlace your fingers to further stretch your pectorals. Option: stand or bend your knees and slowly hinge from your hips into a bent-knee Forward Fold, resting your belly on your thighs. Raise your hands toward the sky with your shoulders down and back.

● **Holding the Pose:** Expand through your chest and lift through your heart center.

● **Modifications:** Stay upright or use a strap between the hands if shoulder flexibility is limited.

STANDING BACK BEND

● **Benefit of the pose:** Another valuable energizer, standing back bends allow you to experience back bends in a particularly safe way, as you can really contract your glutes and extend out of your lower back. This pose will strengthen your glutes and lower back and stretch your chest, shoulders, hip flexors, and abdominals. This pose will also improve flexibility in your spine.

● **Getting into the Pose:** Move slowly. Firm your glutes and place your hands or fists on the bony points alongside your spine. Push your hips forward and lift your chest to the sky.

● **Holding the Pose:** Lift out of your lower back, drawing your elbows back to expand your chest. Without dropping your head back, look up toward the sky.

● **Modifications:** People recovering from a lower back injury should use caution. Use Standing Chest Expansion as an alternative, if necessary. If your neck fatigues, look forward, tucking your chin slightly.

WARRIOR I

● **Benefit of the pose:** Tap into your warrior spirit with this powerful pose. This pose is part of the Warrior series. Benefits include increased physical and mental strength, enhanced power, and determination. Warrior I strengthens the quads, glutes, lats, upper back, and shoulders.

● **Getting into the Pose:** From Mountain pose, step back into a short stance and align your heels. Bend your front knee, stacking it over your ankle. Straighten your back leg, turning your toes slightly forward. Square your hips and shoulders with the front of your mat. Raise your arms to the sky.

● **Holding the Pose:** Continue to press the outer edge of your back foot into the mat. Open your hands and activate your fingers. Relax your shoulders and point your tailbone straight down. Engage your abs as you lift up with your upper body and sink into your forward leg. Keep your forward knee over your ankle. Switch sides.

● **Modifications:** To decrease the intensity, straighten the forward leg slightly or shorten your stance. In the event of shoulder discomfort, bring your hands to prayer position.

WARRIOR II

● **Benefit of the pose:** Warrior II is an excellent strengthener for your lower body and shoulders. This is an excellent pose to enhance focus, determination, and warrior spirit. This powerful pose strengthens the quads and shoulders and creates core stabilization. In this pose, you will focus on moving energy outward while turning your awareness inward for strength, focus, and discipline.

● **Getting into the Pose:** From Warrior I, keep your heels aligned as you open your hips and shoulders to the long edge of your mat. Lower your arms parallel to the floor, reaching out in opposite directions through your fingers. Keep your front knee bent and your hips level. Look over your front hand.

● **Holding the Pose:** Lift your upper body and reach through your fingers in opposite directions. Sink through your lower body, keeping your knee over your ankle. Engage your abs and relax your shoulders back and down.

● **Modifications:** To decrease the intensity, straighten the forward leg slightly or shorten your stance. In the event of shoulder discomfort, bring your hands to prayer position.

REVERSE WARRIOR

● **Getting into the Pose:** From Warrior II, turn your front palm up and lift into lateral flexion. Take your back hand to your back leg for support, resting it lightly. Keep your hips squared to the side wall and maintain your Warrior II leg position. Stack the wrist of your front arm over your front shoulder.

● **Holding the Pose:** For Reverse Warrior, retain your Warrior base as you lift strongly towards the sky.

● **Modifications:** You can decrease the distance of your stance if joint discomfort occurs. You can also bend your top arm at the elbow to decrease the lever.

EXTENDED ANGLE

● **Getting into the Pose:** From Warrior II, place your forward forearm on your forward thigh, as you extend your top arm toward the sky for Side Angle. Relax your shoulders away from your ears. Stay here, or reach your forward hand inside the foot and extend your top arm over your ear, palm facing down for Extended Angle. Press the back of your arm against your thigh and your thigh against your arm to revolve your chest open toward the sky. Sink your hips down while pressing them forward.

● **Modifications:** You can shorten your stance or lower your top arm if you experience joint discomfort. You can use a block under your lower hand.

TRIANGLE

● **Benefit of the pose:** This pose is one of my favorite yoga poses. It moves energy in four directions, originating from a strong center. Triangle strengthens the quads, obliques, and shoulders. Triangle also stretches the hamstrings, pectorals, and intercostals.

Your upper body is lifting and moving back while your lower body is sinking and moving forward. Triangle pose represents creating for ourselves a strong mental and physical foundation, represented by the two bottom points of the triangle. From here, you can begin to look up, exploring the third point—the spiritual.

● **Getting into the Pose:** From the Warrior II or Side Angle pose, straighten your front leg. Reach forward, then lower your hand to your shin or ankle. Lift your back arm to the sky, opening your chest. Look up, down, or straight ahead, finding a comfortable place for your neck.

● **Holding the Pose:** Press your feet away from each other, keeping a soft bend in the forward knee. Check that your nose stays over your leg, not in front of it. Engage your glutes. Breathe length into your spine, allowing your inner strength to fuel your outer strength. Switch sides.

● **Modifications:** If your hamstrings are tight, place your hand on a block.

TWISTING LUNGE

● **Benefit of the pose:** Twisting Lunge is a great toner for the internal organs; like all standing and seated twists, it provides a squeeze and soak effect for the internal organs, wringing out the blood and then flushing the organs with fresh blood. This pose will strengthen your quads, hip adductors and abductors, and upper back. It will stretch your hip flexors and obliques. Practice this pose when your body is thoroughly warm.

● **Getting into the Pose:** From a lunge position with your right foot forward, place your left hand on the floor close to your right foot. With a straight spine, sweep your right arm up, reaching toward the sky.

● **Holding the Pose:** Press through your back heel and stack your forward knee over the ankle. Keep your chest close to your forward knee as you twist from the waist. Look up. Switch sides.

● **Modifications:** Drop your back knee to the mat for a Kneeling Lunge. Place your bottom hand on a block to help lengthen the spine for rotation.

● **Take it to the next level:** A variation called the Prayer Twisting Lunge: Do a kneeling lunge, place your hands in prayer position over your heart. Rotate, placing the back of your arm against the outside of your forward thigh. Lift your back knee off the mat and look up for Prayer Twisting Lunge.

PYRAMID

● **Getting into the Pose:** From a short Warrior I stance, square your hips to the front of the mat and anchor your back heel. With your hands at heart center, you're hinging from your hips and leading from the heart center. Straighten your front knee to a comfortable position. Keep a neutral spine and allow your hands to rest where they land, bringing them to your thigh, shin, ankle, or the floor.

● **Modifications:** Bend front knee slightly if there is joint discomfort. Widen stance to hip distance.

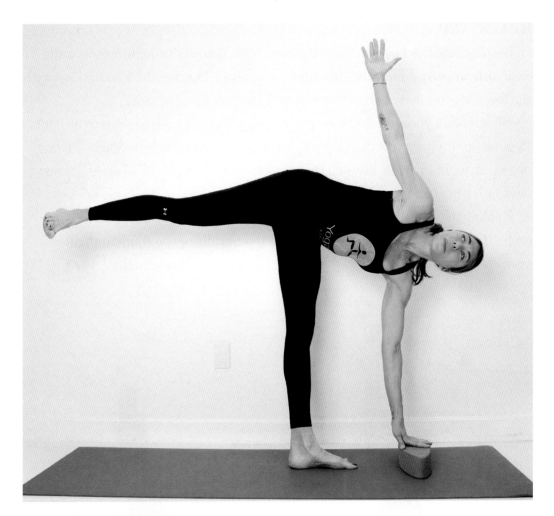

BALANCING HALF MOON

● **Getting into the Pose:** From Pyramid, bend your front knee slightly so you can shift your weight forward onto your front foot, raise your back leg to hip height, push back through your heels, place your right fingertips on the floor (directly under your shoulder), and turn your hips and chest out to the side. Revolve your torso and lift your top ribcage toward the sky. Placing your top hand on our hip, engage your abs and glutes with the option to extend your top arm. Finding a focal point; feel your breath. Continue lengthening from your back heel to the crown of your head, keeping your head in line with your spine. Look down or to the side.

● **Modifications:** Elevating the supporting hand on a block to reduce stretch the hamstring. We can practice the pose with our backs against wall to maintain support in the pose.

HEADSTAND

● **Getting into the Pose:** From "all fours," with your feet touching the wall and your wrists under your shoulders, come into Downward-Facing Dog with the heels of your feet against the wall and your toes on the mat.

Slowly walk your feet halfway up the wall with your legs parallel to the floor. Begin straightening your legs, lifting your hips and extending your arms. Bring one leg straight up while keeping the other foot on the wall. Avoid arching your back or letting your legs fall toward the middle of the room. Do both sides.

● **Holding the Pose:** Relaxing your neck, do not allow your back to sway or arch. If your shoulders are tight, look to the middle of the room and allow your shoulders to rise toward your ears. Keep your arms straight.

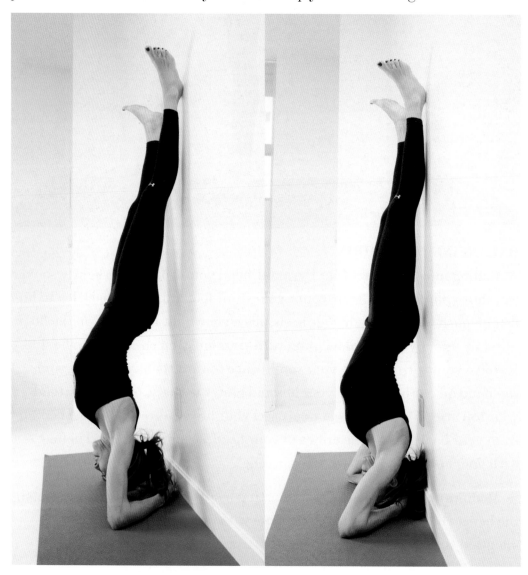

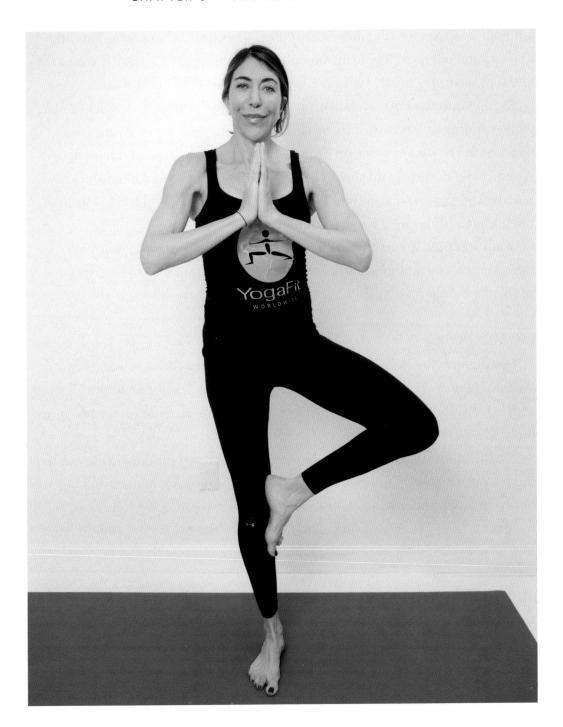

TREE

● **Benefit of the pose:** A powerful standing balance pose, tree will force
you to use all the muscles in your legs and engage your core. This pose
will strengthen your legs, abdominals, and glutes as well as your powers of
concentration. This popular balance pose promotes poise and calm. Visualize

yourself as a tree, rooting down through your standing leg and expanding upward and outward like branches through your arms. Play with your arm and foot positions until you find a steady place to hold and breathe.

● **Getting into the Pose:** Balance on one leg. Bring your opposite foot onto your standing ankle, calf, or inner thigh, avoiding your knee. Bring your hands into the prayer position or raise your arms overhead and look up. Holding the Pose: Lift up through the crown of your head while firmly rooting through your standing foot. Contract your abs and level your hips. Switch sides. Finding a focal point helps.

● **Modifications:** If you have difficulty balancing, place the toes of your raised leg on the mat or stand next to a wall for support. People with knee problems should use caution.

CHILD'S POSE

● **Getting into the Pose:** From all fours, sink your hips back toward your heels and lower your body toward your thighs. Reach your arms out in front of you for Extended Child's Pose or bring your arms around alongside your body. Rest, relaxing and checking in with your body.

● **Modification:** Place a bolster, blanket, or extra mat behind your knees to reduce knee flexion. Cause dorsiflexion of your ankles by resting on your toes or placing mat underneath your ankles to reduce plantar flexion. Rest your head on fists, or your chest on a block. Separate the thighs to provide room for the body.

SUPPORTED CHILD'S POSE

Begin by placing a bolster vertical to the body or using several stacked blankets. From a kneeling position, bend forward to rest entire torso and head on props. Place a rolled up towel or blanket behind knees to reduce knee flexion or build up height of props to that torso is completely supported.

SPINAL BALANCE

● **Benefits of the pose:** Spinal Balance encourages your core center muscles to stabilize as you resist gravity. It also strengthens your glutes, upper and lower back, chest, and shoulders.

● **Getting into the Pose:** From your hands and knees, stabilize your shoulders and hips. Extend one arm out at the height of your shoulder. Lift the opposite leg just to the height of your hips.

● **Holding the Pose:** Keep a long line from your fingers to your heel and hold for five to ten breaths. Focus on stability and strength while you lift your navel to your spine. You may also flow this pose: Inhale as you lengthen your arm and leg and exhale as you bring them back to the floor, then switch sides. Continue to reach forward with your fingers and press back through your heel, toes to the floor, with little or no movement in the torso. Repeat five to ten times per side.

● **Modifications:** To relieve wrist tension, use fists for wrists, palms facing each other. For knee comfort, place padding or make a fold in the mat to kneel on. For less sensation, extend just the arm or just the leg.

CAMEL

● **Benefit of the pose:** This is an amazing opener that is energizing and creates self-confidence and chi flow. It opens the heart center and counteracts the forward flexion that is part of daily living. This pose strengthens the glutes and the lower back as well as stretching pectorals (chest), intercostals, hip flexors, and shoulders. Only do this pose when the body is warmed up, and always follow a back bend with a forward bend.

● **Getting into the Pose:** Move slowly, feeling your way. From a kneeling position, place your hands or fists on the bony points alongside your spine. Firm your glutes. Push your hips forward and lift your chest to the sky. Getting into the Pose: Lift out of your lower back, drawing your elbows back to expand your chest. Look up toward the sky without dropping your head back. As you get out of the pose, go into Child's Pose. Rest.

● **Modifications:** People with lower back issues or injuries should be cautious. Use chest expansion from the knees, if necessary. If your neck fatigues, look forward and tuck your chin slightly. For sensitive knees or another knee issue, use padding.

● **Take it to the next level:** Curl your toes under. Drop your arms behind you and grab your heels. Or, for a bigger challenge, place the tops of your feet on the mat.

CAT AND COW

● **Benefit of the pose:** These two poses are excellent energy builders as they move energy stuck in the lower back and midsection. Flow this pose with the breath to warm up the torso and spine. Benefits include strengthening of abdominal, upper back, lower back, and chest muscles.

● **Getting into the Pose:** From hands and knees, assume the Cat pose—create a C shape with your spine, bringing the heart center toward the tailbone and round your middle back toward the sky. Moving into Cow, create a C shape with your spine, but in the other direction. Pull the heart center away from the tailbone, lifting the crown of your head to the sky. Stack shoulders over wrists, hips over knees. Hold the pose for five deep breaths in each direction.

● **Modifications:** Use fists to prevent hyperextension issues with your wrist. For sensitive knees and knee issues, use extra padding.

DOWNWARD FACING DOG

● **Benefit of the pose:** This pose opens you across your chest and helps you breathe fully through your abdomen. It opens the front of your shoulders while building shoulder strength. It stretches the whole back of your body, including calves, hamstrings, glutes, and major back muscles. This pose releases tension in the body and, through the inversion affect, aids blood flow to your brain. It creates a sense of alertness to prepare you for what comes next. With regular practice, this pose can also be very restful.

● **Getting into the Pose:** From Child's Pose, tuck your toes under and reach your arms ahead. Press into your toes and spread your fingers wide while you lift your hips to the sky. Make an inverted V shape with your body. Holding the Pose: Inhale to reach your tailbone up and lengthen your spine. Exhale to bring your chest and belly toward your thighs.

● **Modifications:** If you have a hard time keeping your spine from rounding, bend your knees to keep your hips hinged and your spine long. To relieve tension in your wrists, come down onto the forearms with your elbows shoulder-width apart. Child's Pose is also an option for a rest at any time.

PLANK

● **Benefit of the pose:** This pose strengthens your entire body. Using good posture techniques as you would when standing, you are now holding your weight above the ground. It strengthens the shoulder chest, lower back, core, glutes, hamstrings, quads, and even muscles in the hands, wrists, feet, and ankles. With the leg extension, you intensify the work in your core center and upper body, and it targets the glute and hamstring of your raised leg. Holding the leg lift can strengthen a swimmer's kick.

● **Getting into the Pose:** From Downward Facing Dog, shift forward so that your shoulders are directly above your wrists. Lengthen your legs and position your pelvis to create a smooth, straight line from your ankles to the crown of your head. With a flexed foot, lift one leg from the hip and keep your pelvis level and your spine long.

● **Holding the Pose:** Lift your belly button to your spine and reach through the crown of your head. Use breath and dynamic tension to spread the work through the entire body.

● **Modifications:** If your lower back drops or your shoulders are up around your ears, choose Kneeling Plank. This will ease tension and reduce the workload while you develop upper body strength.

CROCODILE

● **Getting into the Pose:** From Plank, shift forward with your toes, bringing your shoulders over your fingertips. From there, exhale and lower your body down until your shoulders, elbows, hips, and heels align. Use your triceps to hover above the floor, elbows hugging your ribcage.

● **Modifications:** Using Kneeling Crocodile if you have wrist issues.

COBRA

● **Benefit of the pose:** This pose strengthens your upper back when lifting. They also strengthen your core center and lower back extensors while stretching your chest and shoulders. Cobra prepares you for more intense back work, while Upward Facing Dog is the more intense option, focusing on your shoulders.

● **Getting into Cobra:** From Plank or Kneeling Plank, bring your body to the floor and keep your hands under your shoulders. Engage your inner thighs and pelvic floor and draw your belly button to your spine. Pull your shoulder blades toward your spine and reach through the crown of your head while you lift your chest and shoulders off of the mat.

● **Holding the Pose:** Continue to lengthen from head to toe while you lift your navel toward your spine and draw your shoulders back and down. In Cobra, instead of pushing up with your hands, let your back muscles lift you up.

● **Modifications:** Feel free to rest back in Child's Pose if this brings on fatigue.

UPWARD FACING DOG

● **Getting into the Pose:** From Crocodile, pull forward from your heart and core. Straighten your arms and come onto the tops of your feet with your knees off the floor for Upward Facing Dog. Push the floor away with your hands and draw your shoulders away from your ears; only the palms of your hands and the tops of our feet are on the mat.

● **Holding the Pose:** Press away from your mat to support your weight and continue to pull your heart forward.

● **Modifications:** Practice Cobra to honor wrists and lower back or to focus on building upper back strength.

KNEELING COBRA

● **Getting into the Pose:** From Kneeling Crocodile, lower your pelvis down to the floor, lifting your chest off the floor and lengthening from the middle and upper back for Cobra. Using your hands to stabilize the body with little or no weight in your hands; emphasizing the work in your back muscles.

KNEELING LUNGE

● **Getting into the Pose:** From Child's Pose, inhale, stepping one foot forward between your hands (using one hand to guide the foot forward, as necessary) while keeping your back knee on the floor in a kneeling position. Lifting one hand at a time to the top of your thigh as you begin to lift your chest is an option.

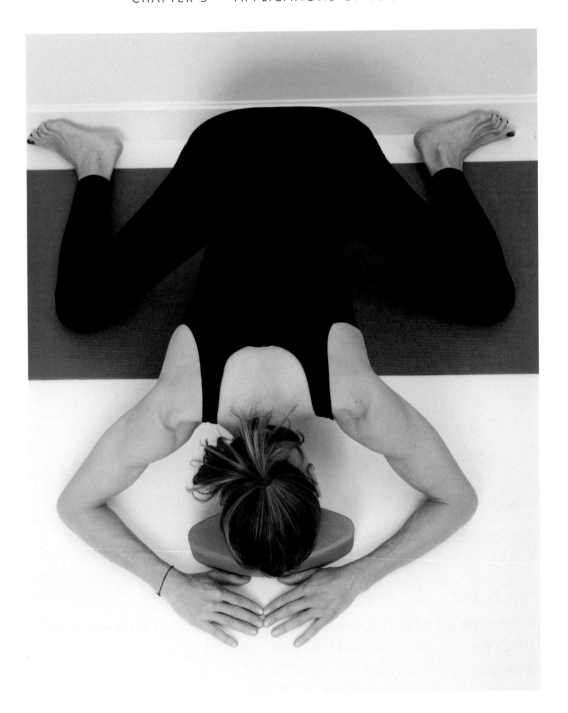

FROG

● **Getting into the Pose:** Beginning in "all fours" pose, separate your knees (out to the side) while bringing your upper body down toward the floor. Keep your hips in line with your knees, lowering your chest and sinking your navel towards the floor. Keep your spine neutral. Keep your abdominals firm.

● **Modifications:** For more stretch, move your knees further apart.

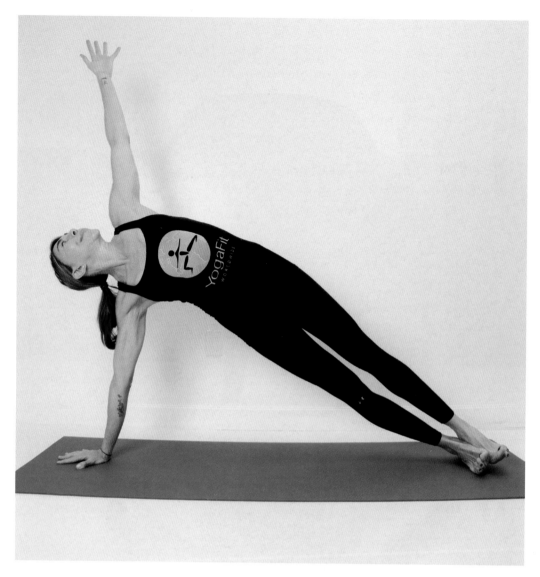

SIDE PLANK

● **Benefit of the pose:** This exercise strengthens your upper body and works to stabilize your shoulders and your core center. Through the rotation, it also strengthens your obliques.

● **Getting into the Pose:** From Plank, stabilize your shoulders, making sure that they are directly over your wrists. Lift one arm up and open into Side Plank. Use your oblique muscles to lift your hip to the sky while you reach further with your arm. Take your raised arm and reach it down and under you while you stay lifted in your hips. Lift your arm back up and repeat.

● **Modifications:** If this exercise is too intense on the shoulders, Kneeling Side Plank will decrease intensity.

KNEELING SIDE PLANK

● **Getting into the Pose:** Begin in Plank Pose, drawing your right knee forward and placing it directly under your right hip with your right foot directly behind your knee. Then extend your left foot out toward the edge of your mat. From here, lift your left arm to the sky. The right hand, right knee, and left foot are all in one line. Your straight leg is supportive, with the ankle flexed and foot pressed into the floor.

● **Modifications:** Use fists for wrists if there is discomfort.

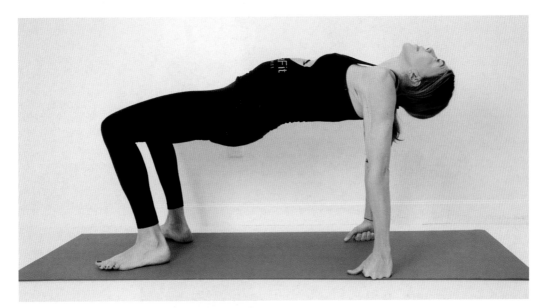

TABLE TOP

● **Benefit of the pose:** Both of these poses strengthen your glutes, hamstrings, inner thighs, rear shoulders, triceps, and your core center. They also stretch the front of your shoulders, chest, and hip flexors.

Getting into Incline Plank: From a seated position, place your hands directly under your shoulders, fingers pointing toward your feet. Pull your shoulder blades back and open your chest. Reach your legs long on your mat with your feet hip distance apart. Press into your heels and lift your hips to the sky. Create a long line between your feet and the crown of your head.

● **Getting into Table Top:** Bend your knees and place your feet flat on your mat. Press your feet into your mat and lift your hips to the sky.

● **Holding the Pose:** In Incline Plank, gently roll your feet inward to prevent your legs from rolling out. In Table Top, you're engaging your inner thighs to align your knees over your ankles. Keep your gaze up without dropping your head back.

● **Modifications:** If you want to relieve tension in your hips and lower back, choose Table Top. If you want to relieve tension in your shoulders, choose Incline Plank. To relieve tension in your hips and shoulders, keep your hips down and stay lifted in your chest and shoulders, or you can lower yourself down to your mat and lift just the hips into Bridge (p. x).

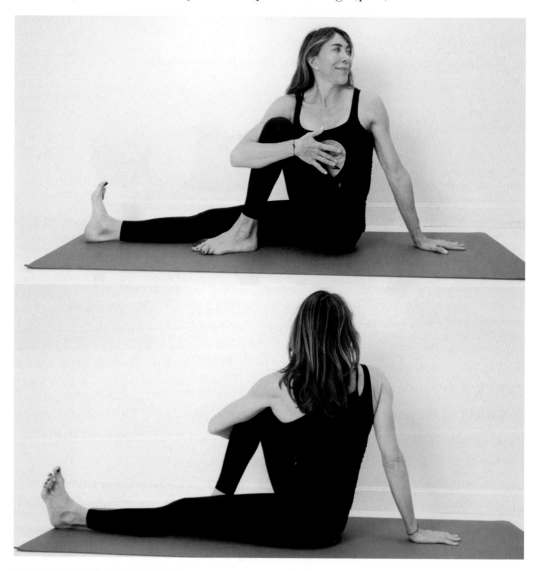

SEATED SPINAL TWIST

● **Getting into the Pose:** While maintaining a neutral spine, bring your right knee in toward your right sitting bone, placing your foot on the floor in line with your sitting bone. Rest your right hand behind you under your shoulder as you lengthen your spine for a twist. Begin your twist by first turning at the navel, then the ribcage, then the upper chest. As you rotate, bring your left forearm around to hold your right shin. Draw your right shoulder blade toward your spine to help deepen your twist. Continue to rest lightly on your right hand while actively pressing through your left heel, toes toward the ceiling.

● **Modifications:** If neutral spine cannot be maintained, sit in a comfortable cross-legged position and twist by bringing left hand to right knee and right hand behind for support.

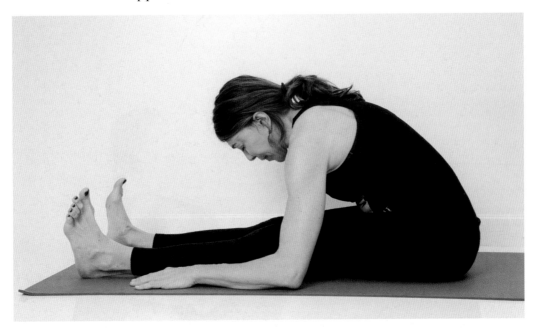

SEATED FORWARD FOLD

● **Benefit of the pose:** Forward folds are cooling and relaxing poses. Over eighty percent of Americans experience some lower back discomfort in their lifetimes. Holding and breathing in forward folds will not only help lengthen your tight hamstrings and lower back muscles, it will also relax you, combating the harmful effects of stress on your mind and body. Anytime you are holding a forward bend or when your head is moving toward the earth (as in Downward Dog), breathe deeply. Focus on completing your exhale and elongating and releasing muscles from the back of your legs, up your spine, perhaps even to that tight place between your ears.

● **Getting into the Pose:** From a seated position, extend your legs. Pull your toes back toward your body. Reach forward, placing your hands on your legs, ankles, feet, or the floor. Using your abs, draw forward through the top of your head.

● **Holding the Pose:** Using a sinking breath, continue to lengthen through your heart and head. Firm your quads. Relax your shoulders back and down. Enjoy the stretch.

● **Modifications:** For tight hamstrings, sit on a folded blanket or a rolled-up yoga mat, use a strap or towel around your feet, or bend your knees.

Take it to the next level: Bend one knee, bringing your foot flat to the floor, toes pointing forward. Keeping your knee pointing straight up, reach forward.

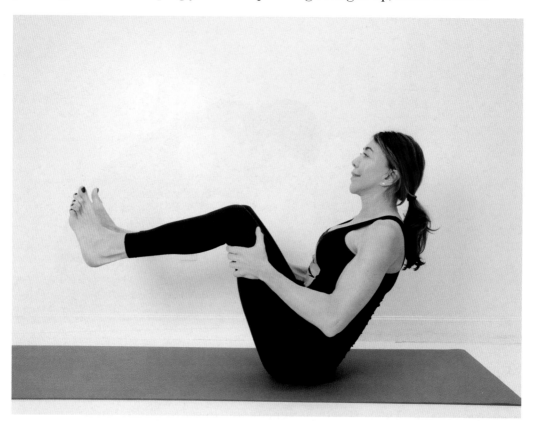

BOAT

● **Benefit of the pose:** Boat pose is an amazing core strengthener, because it activates your power center. Boat pose also helps engage your core muscles. Boat pose strengthens the abdominals, hip flexors, and quadriceps as well as targeting the back muscles. The pose strengthens the core and improves balance.

● **Getting into the Pose:** Sitting upright on the floor, bend your knees and hold onto your hamstrings. Slowly lift one foot at a time away from the floor, keeping your back straight. Reach forward with your arms as you balance on the back of your glutes.

● **Holding the Pose:** Focus on your breath to lengthen your spine and lift your chest, relaxing your shoulders backward and down.

● **Modifications:** If you have back injuries or are a beginner, keep your feet on the floor and continue holding your hamstrings.

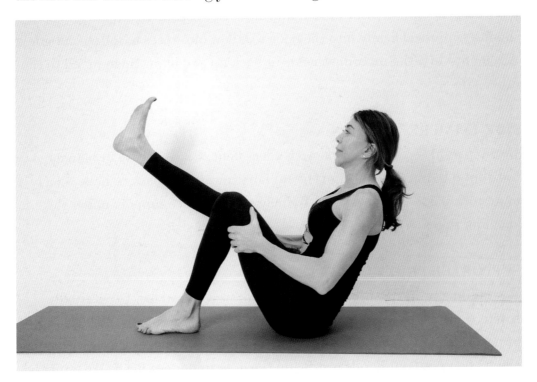

● **Take it to the next level:** Straighten your legs and reach forward without rounding your back.

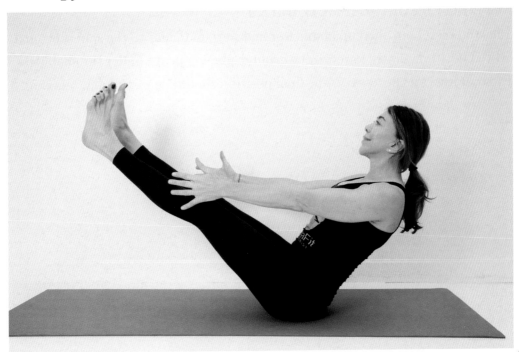

WINDSHIELD WIPERS

From a supine position, we are bending our knees, placing the soles of our feet on the floor. Our arms are extended out to the sides in a T. Keeping our shoulders pressed firmly into the floor, we allow our knees to fall to one side. After a few breaths, we bring the knees back up and allow them to fall to the other side.

SIDE-LYING RELAXATION

Begin in a side-seated position with knees bent. Place bolster or blanket horizontal to hip, with most of the support toward the back or hips. Slowly lower into a side-lying position. We may need to place support under the shoulder to reach the floor.

SUPPORTED PRONE OR BELLY

Lay flat in a prone position on the floor. Allow legs and feet to externally rotate. Place a rolled up blanket or small bolster underneath the belly, hips, or pelvic region. We have the option of placing our arms overhead with our elbows bent and our hands resting on the floor under our head. We want the entire body to feel relaxed and at ease in this pose.

SUPPORTED CORPSE OR *SAVASANA*

Place a bolster or rolled up blanket or mat perpendicular to the spine. From a seated position, slowly lower to the ground, placing props under the shoulders, torso, or knees as necessary. The final position should be restful and relaxing.

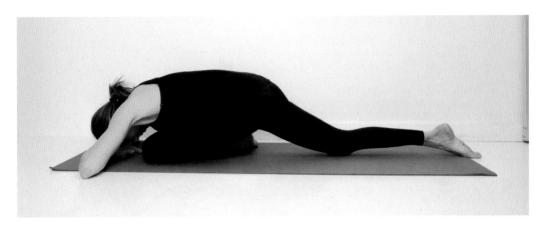

PIGEON

● **Benefit of the pose:** Great for releasing tension and stress, Pigeon stretches the deep glute muscles in the back of the hips. It also helps to stretch the band of muscle that runs down the outside of the thigh from the hip to the knee that gets tight with a lot of running (IT Band).

● **Getting into the Pose:** From Downward Facing Dog, bring one leg forward to the floor with your knee bent and your foot flexed. Stay lifted enough to keep your pelvis level.

● **Holding the Pose:** Release your upper body down to the floor and rest your forehead on your hands or stacked fists.

● **Modifications:** To make this pose more restorative, lie on your back with your knees bent and your feet on the floor. Lift one leg and place your foot on your other thigh for support. Reach to hold the supporting leg behind the knee and draw your leg in toward your chest. If your range of motions allows, Standing Pigeon from Chair Pose is another option. Bring one ankle to the top of the opposite thigh with your foot flexed and sit back into Chair

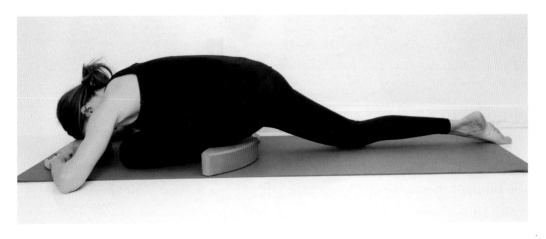

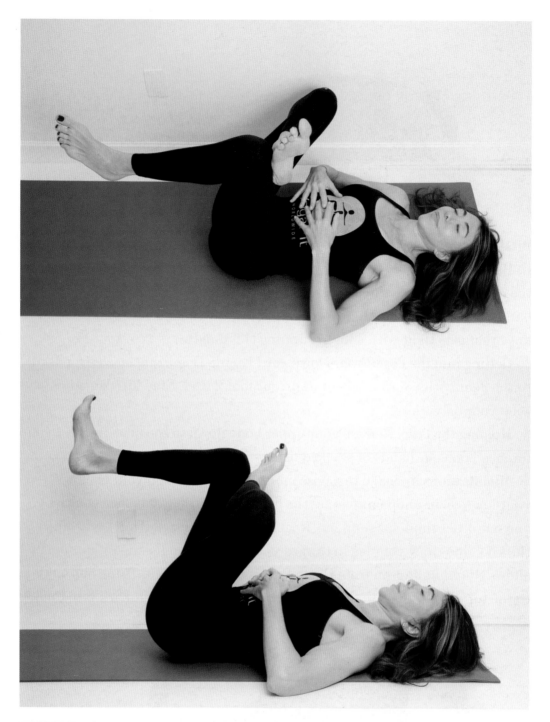

FIGURE FOUR

● **Getting into the Pose:** Lying down on your back, bring both knees in toward your chest, crossing one knee over the other. Reaching behind the thigh of the uncrossed leg, gently pull the leg toward your chest while maintaining neutral spine. Switch legs and repeat.

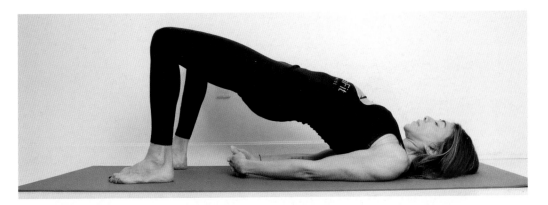

BRIDGE

● **Benefit of the pose:** Bridge pose is an excellent way to stretch the front of the hips and open your chest, particularly if you sit for long periods or regularly walk, run, or cycle. Many people have tight hip flexors from too much walking, running, cycling, or even just sitting or driving. Bridge pose also targets muscles deep in the lower back and hips that are difficult to reach when upright. This pose will strengthen your glutes, hamstrings, adductors, and abductors. Bridge will stretch your hip flexors, core center, and pectorals.

● **Getting into the Pose:** Lie down on your back, palms down. Slide your shoulders away from your ears. Bring the soles of your feet to the floor, hip-width apart. Press through your feet to lift your hips.

● **Holding the Pose:** Keep your head still to protect your neck—don't look around. Use your inner thighs to keep your knees in line with your hips and toes. Breathe deeply into your open chest and naval center.

● **Modifications:** Turn the palms up for more chest opening and core focus.

● **Take it to the next level:** Interlace your fingers under your body. Walk your shoulders toward each other so that your body is resting on the outside edges

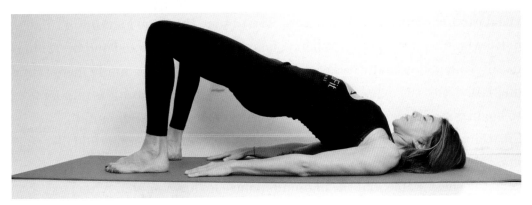

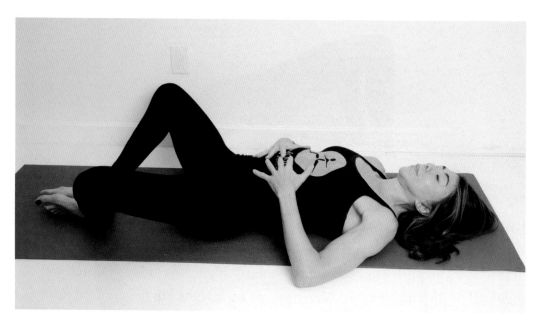

RECLINING BUTTERFLY

● **Benefit of the pose:** Use Reclining Butterfly after your body is warmed during Mountain 3 to strengthen your abs and hip flexors. It will also stretch your hips, glutes, and lower back.

● **Getting into the Pose:** Lying down with a straight spine, place the soles of your feet together in front of you. Let your knees drop open, and the weight of gravity will stretch your adductors and hip flexors. Use your outer thighs to draw your knees toward the floor.

BELLY BREATHING

● **Getting into the Pose:** Lying on the back is the optimal place for learning belly breathing. First, place the right hand on the chest and the left hand on the upper part of the abdomen, then breathe so that the left hand moves up on the inhalation and the right hand remains virtually motionless. On the exhalation, the left hand then lowers. Try to take the same amount of time both exhaling and inhaling. When you are completely relaxed and breathing nasally and abdominally, it is easier to inhale evenly and to fluidly merge the inhalation into the exhalation. For the smoothest transition, it is important to begin your inhale consciously, just as the exhale ends. Abdominal breathing in final relaxation pose is the simplest and easiest method of breathing. The diaphragm is active, the intercostal muscles act mainly to keep the chest stable, and the abdominal muscles are completely relaxed.

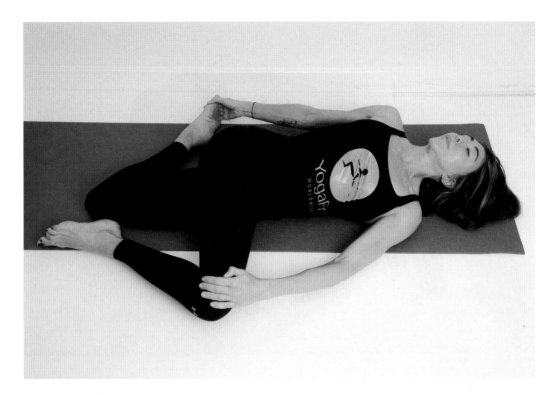

SPINAL TWIST

● **Benefit of the pose:** This pose will help you stretch out your lower back and open up your thoracic spine. From a lying position you can lengthen your spine with ease because you don't need to work against gravity. The twist invigorates your torso muscles, stimulates conductivity of your sensory nerves, and massages your internal organs.

● **Getting into the Pose:** Lie on the mat on your back and bring your right knee to a bent position with your foot on the floor beside your left leg. Press into your foot and lift your pelvis up enough to shift your pelvis to the right and then rest it on the floor. Keep your right shoulder on the mat and use your left hand to gently draw your right knee over left and toward the floor.

● **Holding the pose:** Keep both shoulders placed on the mat and look over your left shoulder to maximize the benefit of the twist. Practice releasing toward the floor with every exhale, then switch sides.

● **Modifications:** From a side-lying position, rotate your upper body open, keeping your hips facing the side. Place a block or two under your right knee or a rolled-up mat lengthwise behind you for support. If you have any disc injuries, this may aggravate the injury. In this case, start with both knees bent and allow both legs to go to one side.

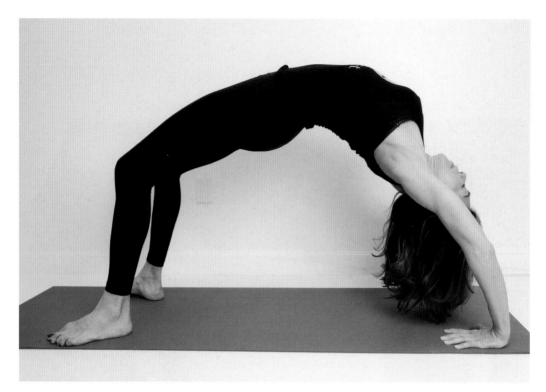

WHEEL

● **Getting into the Pose:** From Bridge pose, place both of your hands on either side of your ears with your fingers pointing toward your feet. Pressing downward evenly with both hands, keep your elbows in line with your wrists, lifting your shoulders and your head off the floor.

● **Holding the pose:** Keep your feet parallel hip distance apart and your weight over your heels until your arms are extended. Keeping your arms strong, slowly extend your legs being mindful of your lower back. Relax your head and neck; working but avoiding straining. Stretch the front of your body longer and longer.

● **Modifications:** Staying in Bridge pose, keep your elbows bent coming up onto the top of your head. Keep the weight on your hands and feet rather than on your head and neck. Do push-ups, raising the hips higher with each consecutive breath. Working slowly and building strength.

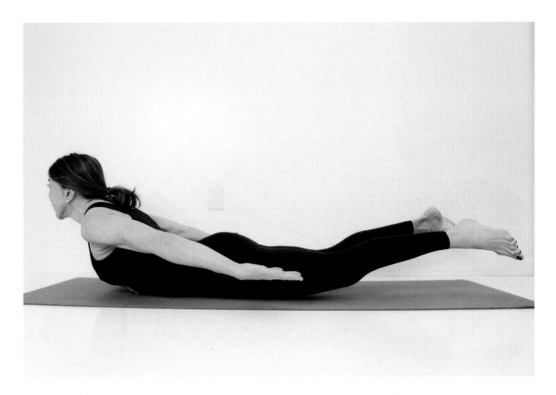

LOCUST

● **Benefit of the pose:** This pose strengthens the entire back of the body, including your hamstrings, glutes, back extensors, upper back, and rear shoulder muscles. It also prepares you for more intense back work in poses like Bow and Camel.

● **Getting into the Pose:** Lie face-down and turn one cheek to the floor with your arms to your sides. Reach with your toes and activate your inner thighs and core center, lifting your belly away from the floor. Reach your shoulder blades toward your spine, lifting your chest and shoulders away from your mat, and let your head follow. Keep your palms facing inward and reach your fingers toward your feet.

● **Holding the Pose:** Maintain a good connection through your core center to protect your lower back. Imagine that you are stretched like a hammock and continue to reach your toes and head away, spreading the work throughout your body.

● **Modifications:** For less sensation, bring your hands back to the floor under your shoulders, as in Cobra, for more support. For more sensation, lift your legs away from the floor, keeping your feet together.

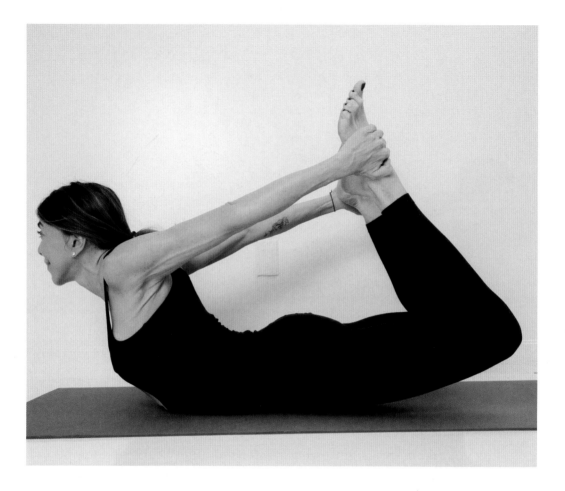

BOW

● **Benefit of the pose:** Bow opens up the whole front side of the body—quads, hip flexors, abdominals, chest, and shoulders—while strengthening the entire back side of the body, including your hamstrings, glutes, back extensors, and upper back. Performed with intense levels of exertion, it helps the body to release tension and pent-up energy. This pose is great for offsetting excessive amounts of forward flexion (rounding of the spine and shoulders).

● **Getting into the Pose:** Lie on your belly and open your shoulders to reach behind to your ankles. Flex your feet and draw your thighs inward. Press your ankles into your hands and hold your ankles firmly. Engage your core center and lift away from the body.

● **Holding the Pose::** Keep a strong core center and continue to lift through the crown of your head and press your ankles into your hands.

● **Modifications:** If you have difficulty getting both hands to your ankles, use Half Bow, which is performed one side at a time. Place one arm in front

of you bent at the elbow. Use your hand and forearm across your mat for
support and reach your other hand to the ankle on the same side. Another
option is to place a strap around your ankle and hold on to the strap.

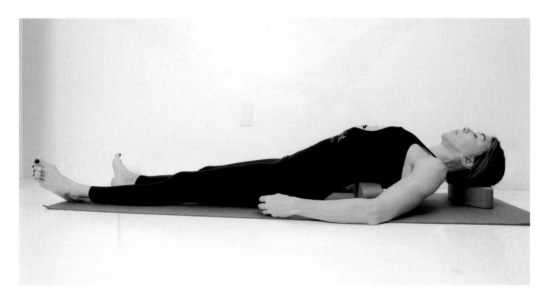

SUPPORTED FISH

● **Benefit of the pose:** Fish pose opens you across your chest and shoulders.
The contour shape of the eggs fully supports your spine in an extended
position. With this support, the body can be at rest for a more restorative
approach.

● **Getting into the Pose:** From a seated position, place three egg blocks
together behind you. Roll onto the rounded edge of the blocks with your
upper back, not your lower back. Extend your legs along your mat and
release your arms out to your sides in a comfortable position.

● **Holding the Pose:** With each exhale, release tension and become more and
more relaxed. Enjoy the stillness.

● **Modifications::** If your neck feels too extended, place another egg block
under your head.

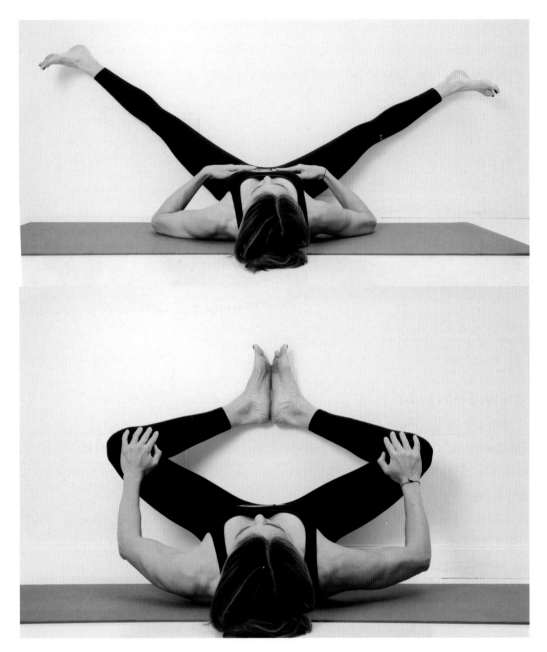

LEGS UP AGAINST WALL

● **Benefit of the pose:** In this inversion, it is hard not to relax. To add a deep, relaxing stretch, play with different leg positions, like Straddle Splits or Butterfly (soles of the feet together, knees open). This will stretch your glutes and hamstrings; if your legs are apart, it will also stretch your hips.

● **Getting into the Pose:** Bring your mat to a wall. From Knees to Chest pose, roll over onto one side until your gluteals are touching the wall. Use your hands to roll onto your back, straightening your legs up the wall.

● **Holding the Pose:** Separate your legs slightly to breathe more easily into the bottom of your lungs.

● **Modifications:** Ask your doctor which inversions are appropriate for you. If no wall is available, make fists and place them under your hips for support.

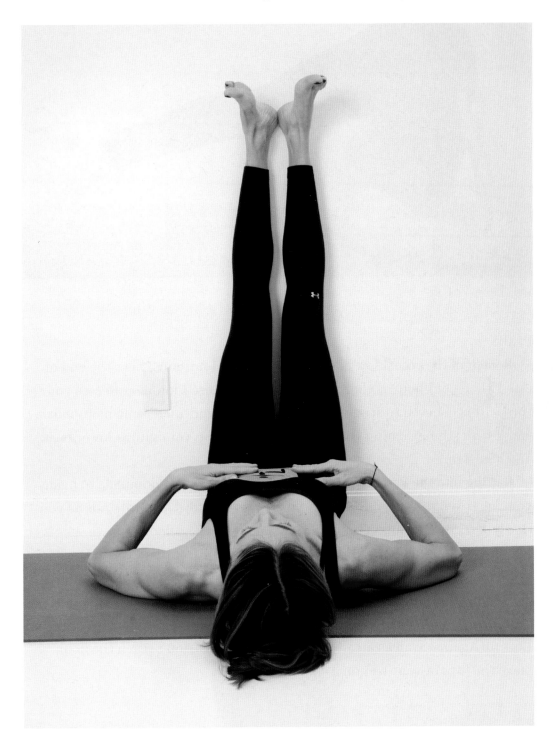

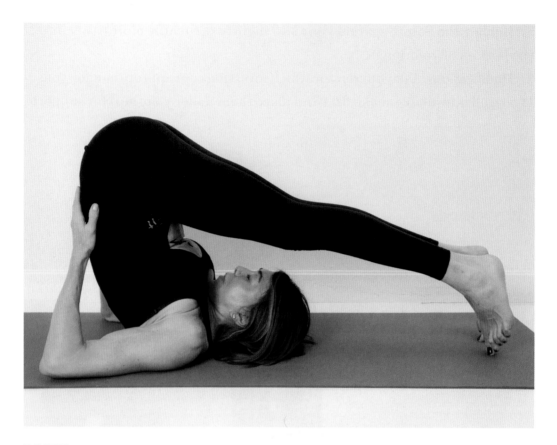

PLOW

● **Benefit of the pose:** Plow is most effective in Mountain 3 near the end of class, when your body is thoroughly warm. Because Plow compresses your throat, it is believed to stimulate your thyroid gland, increasing metabolism, along with strengthening your abs while stretching your glutes, lower back, and hamstrings.

● **Getting into the Pose:** Lying on your back, use your abdominals to bring your legs over your head. Support your lower back with your hands as you slowly straighten your legs and place your toes on the floor.
Holding the Pose: Keep your legs straight. If your feet don't touch the floor, support your lower back with your hands. Breathe into your throat.

● **Modifications:** People with certain conditions should not attempt this pose. Ask your doctor which inversions are appropriate for you. Practice Legs up Against Wall as an alternative. If your toes don't reach the floor, place the tops of your feet on a chair.

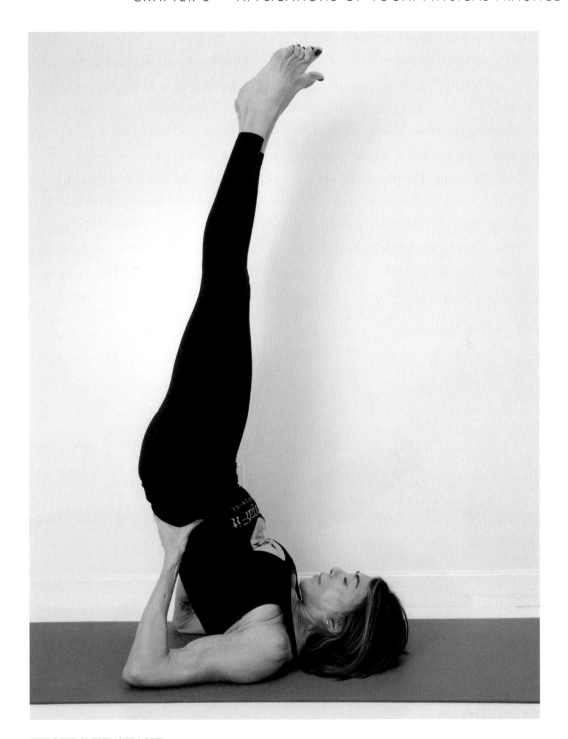

SHOULDER STAND

● **Benefit of the pose:** Shoulder Stand is an inversion that follows the Plow pose at the end of Mountain 3. Like Plow, this pose is believed to stimulate the thyroid gland, increasing metabolism. Always follow with Knees to Chest pose, and it will strengthen your upper and lower back, abs, and glutes, while stretching your shoulders and chest.

● **Getting into the Pose:** From Plow pose, bend your knees and support your back with your hands as you lift your legs to the sky. Don't move your head or neck.

● **Holding the Pose:** Keep a slight bend at the waist and knees for less pressure on your neck. Breathe into your throat.

● **Modifications:** People with certain conditions should not attempt this pose. Ask your doctor which inversions are appropriate for you. Practice Legs up Against Wall as an alternative.

● **Take it to the next level:** Straighten your legs and continue lifting them to the sky until your body is perpendicular to the floor. For less pressure on your neck, keep a slight bend at the waist. Don't move your head or neck.

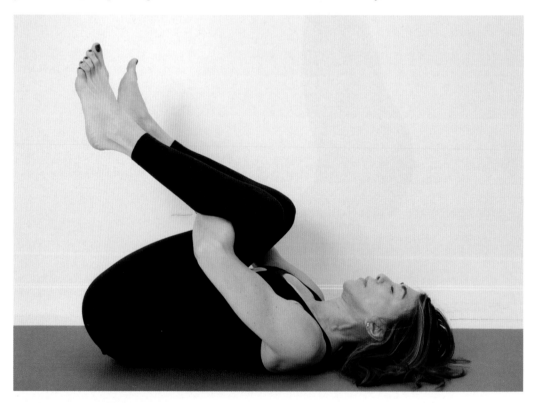

KNEES TO CHEST

● **Getting into the Pose:** From a supine position, we're drawing our knees into our chest, holding our legs behind our thighs. For a light back massage, rock gently from side to side.

● **Modifications:** Use a towel or strap to reach around the thighs if there is limited hip flexion

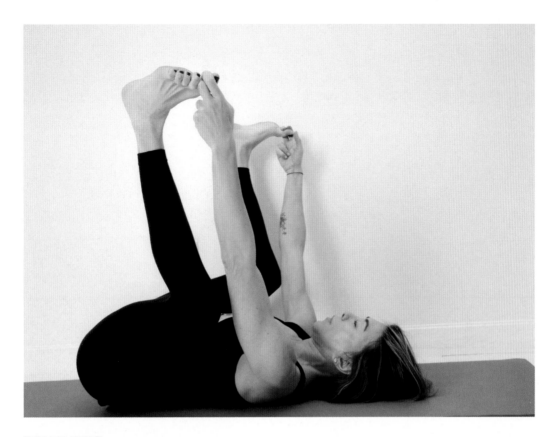

DEAD BUG

● **Benefit of the pose:** For this pose, allow yourself to feel supported by gravity as you release physical and emotional tension from your back and hips. Practice this pose near the end of Mountain 3, before inversions, and it will strengthen your biceps while stretching your hips and glutes.

● **Getting into the Pose:** From Knees to Chest pose, hold your hamstrings and draw your knees down toward the floor. If your tailbone is resting on the floor, lift the soles of your feet toward the sky. If your tailbone lifts off the floor, keep your knees bent.

● **Holding the Pose:** Bring your elbows out to each side; as you continue, draw your knees toward the floor. Rest your head, shoulders, and tailbone on the floor as you stretch.

● **Modifications:** If Dead Bug is uncomfortable, stay in Knees to Chest pose. Take it to the next level: Grab your big toes with your index and middle fingers and draw your knees toward the floor. Keep your ankles stacked over your knees.

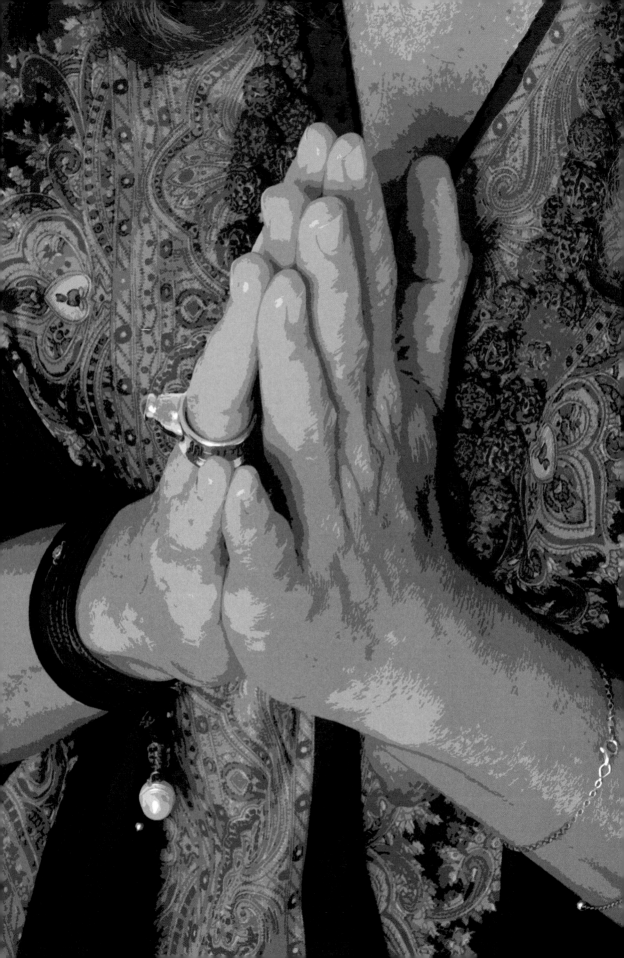

CHAPTER 6

Applications of Yoga: Meditation

"As a lamp in a windless place does not waver, so the yogi whose mind is focused remains always steady in meditation on the transcendent Self."
—BHAGAVAD GITA 6:19

"Yoga is calming the fluctuations of the mind."
—YOGA SUTRAS 1:2

Meditation saves my life often. Despite enjoying yoga, fitness, health, a great career, many friends, and the rest of the beautiful things in my life, at times, I suffer from depression. I have even considered suicide a few times in my life. Whether by nature or nurture, I am a highly sensitive person who experiences fluctuations of moods that are, by and large, positive due to a very disciplined, and at times rigorous, practice of all the tools in this book. You may be surprised to read this, and believe me I'm even more surprised to put this in print, but for anyone who has suffered trauma, chances are they have had similar experiences. When the going gets tough, I don't turn to alcohol, drugs, or food. I exercise, do yoga, and meditate. Some days I need to meditate twice a day: usually silent or mantra in the morning, guided late afternoon. Sometimes I'll even sleep with the *Bhagavad Gita* playing in the background. Because I'm so physically active—yoga, exercise, and lots of travel—I find meditation to be incredibly balancing, grounding, and centering.

Meditation is a force in transforming your psyche, your soul, and your mind and body. My goal is to introduce you to different types of meditation so that you can try them all and see what works best for you. The road to healing has many paths, and we must all find the one that works best for us. Even more important, I believe, is the willingness to walk down many.

Try different techniques to see which one works for you and even if you don't think you're succeeding at it, do it anyway. Start by finding one or two ideal times per day and schedule around that. Yoga Bhajan said it takes forty days to make or break a habit. Try committing to forty days to make that habit stick. Be easy on yourself if you miss a day; it's ok.

Meditation can have a profound effect on the health of those who practice regularly. Meditation has been found to lower blood pressure, improve immune function, significantly lower stress hormone release (including cortisol), lower oxygen consumption, decrease feelings of anxiety and depression, improve sleep, and decrease chronic pain, just to name a few of the studied benefits. There are many types of meditation including, prayer, guided imagery, progressive relaxation, Transcendental Meditation (TM), Zen Buddhist meditation, Japa, movement meditation, mindfulness meditation, Yoga *nidra*, medical meditation, and more. Let's start with the proper meditation space set up for those dealing with trauma, PTSD, depression, and anxiety.

Prior to beginning your meditation journey, create a space that works for you. For some, it will be a darkened room; for others, bright daylight. You must feel safe in your space. As I mentioned in my book *YogaLean*, the first space I ever set up to meditate when I lived at the beach in my early twenties was literally the former trash closet in my kitchen. Obviously, depending on one's trauma background, this would be less than ideal for some and a more open room would work better. The room shape and configuration and the surrounding environment is important to consider when creating a safe place for release and healing.

You can sit in a comfortable position with your spine straight, be it in a chair or directly on the floor. You can also lie down, which is particularly good for guided meditation. If you are not comfortable, you will be distracted. If you are meditating before or after your yoga practice, roll up your mat and sit on it, as elevating your hips eases tension in the hips and hamstrings and improves circulation to your legs. You may want additional props like blocks, blankets, and bolsters. As in the YogaFit SPA principles, we listen to the body and let go of judgement and the idea that there is a perfect meditation pose. You may want to use headphones or earplugs to block out ambient noise. I also love to use essential oils in a diffuser to help create the space, I find lavender and rosemary especially healing.

If you have been through trauma, ideally your room is calm, quiet and out of the way. Sometimes your meditation space can be in your head, like mine was when I was six years old and I would visualize myself on a beach or in the forest. When I meditate now, I like to envision an all grey room, this feels peaceful, safe, and calm for me.

Meditation may prove challenging to some trauma survivors. Someone who has experienced trauma or abuse may be triggered by a scene described in visualization, for example. Trauma survivors are likely to be disconnected from their bodies and from the world around them. Meditations that keep the focus on the body and breath such as chanting, yoga *nidra*, or progressive relaxation may be less likely to trigger someone than a meditation such as mindfulness meditation wherein the participant is encouraged to let the mind wander. Many trauma survivors are hypervigilant, and it may feel safer for some people to keep their eyes wide open. Keeping the lights on but lowered, if possible, may be a good solution.

For those of us who suffer from trauma, meditation becomes a life saver, and a lifeline. Meditation can be healing, clearing, and simultaneously connecting. I find that the feelings I get from meditation truly surpass all worldly experiences. As a trauma survivor, meditation is one of the things that helps us become "thrivers." Active meditation involves focusing our brain's energy and awareness on a particular thought or visualization. Attempting to clear and focus our minds can help us to temporarily calm and give space to emotions and thoughts that do not serve us. While the styles of meditation differ, the end goal is the same: the Three Cs—calm, connection, and clarity—all being used primarily to engage in relaxation. Whatever your meditation practice looks like, however, be sure to embrace the essence of YogaFit: Let go of all judgment of your experience.

There are four styles of meditation, which I like to call The Four Ss—Sound, Sight, Silence, and Somatic. For each one, there are different techniques. One may resonate more than the others, depending on your trauma experience, symptoms, or simply your preference.

Sound—Mantra and Guide-Based Meditation

I love mantra-based meditation because it creates a mental focal point. The repetition of a sound forces us to focus. If our minds are wandering, we then bring them back to the mantra. Ideally it becomes the heartbeat of our meditation. A mantra can be a phrase, a word, a syllable, or a group of words used during meditation. A chant is a rhythmical repetition of a song, sound, phrase, or word. I've been practicing mantra based meditation for seven years now, and it has changed my life.

Mantra-Based

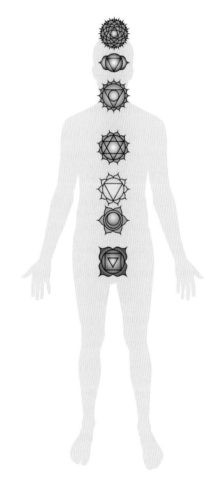

Transformational Chakra Meditation is a YogaFit program designed to be a self-growth tool. It is a healing, anti-aging, stress-reducing technique that incorporates the focuses on the chakras, the body's energy centers. This form of meditation gives us the opportunity to balance ourselves ourselves and our energy. To practice this meditation, simply breathe into all of your energy centers starting with the base of the spine, the root chakra, represented by the color red. Visualize each chakra color getting brighter as you move upward. Do several times for ten minutes anytime you feel out of balance. It is a tool to facilitate deep shifts on an energetic and emotional or physical basis. We teach this at many of YogaFit's Mind Body Fitness Conferences.

Sound Chanting is a great way to start your meditation practice. I like to chant along with my favorite "chantress" Snatam Kaur or Deva Premal. I love "Ra Ma Da Sa Sa Say So Hung/The Siri Gaitri Mantra," chanted by and with Snatam Kaur (Snatam Kaur's CD is available at YogaFit.com). This is a great way to start a mantra-based meditation practice, and it literally saved my life during a very challenging time, alleviating a lot of stress and anxiety. It was the only music I could listen to for a month because of the peace and calm it helped me discover. To this day, when I am stressed out and I feel my heart racing, I turn on this chant and chant along at the top of my lungs until I feel better. It's a real "letting go of judgment" moment allowing myself to tap into the chant with such conviction.

"The Siri Gaitri Mantra" is a *kundalini* yoga healing chant that heals by tuning the soul to the pure vibration of the universe. The words to this mantra are "Ra Ma Da Sa Sa Say So Hung."

Ra means the sun and connecting with that solar energy frequency.

Ma means the moon and aligns us to receive.

Da is the energy of the earth and it grounds us.

Sa is infinity and brings energy up and out drawing to create space for the universe to heal us.

Sa for a second time, pulls the energy of infinity into us.

Say is a way of honoring the all-encompassing energy of the universe.

So is the vibration of the ultimate union.

Hung is the infinite, the vibrating real, and the essence of creation.

(So Hung together means, I am Thou.)

Repeating a mantra either out loud or silently on the exhale can be helpful too. Here are some examples:

- **Sa Ta Na Ma:** Also called the Primordial Sound Mantra because it consists of the five primordial sounds, *S, T, N, M, and ah*. Sa means birth and evokes a sense of emotion and expansiveness. Ta means life and creates transformation and strength. Na means death and evokes a sense of universal love. Ma means rebirth and stimulates communication.
- **Shalom, Shanti.** Peace, Peace
- **Om Mani Padme Hum:** Tibetan mantra meaning, "May the jewel in the lotus of my heart shine brightly connecting all in love and light."

- **Healthy I am, Happy I am, Holy I am:** reminds one that health, happiness, and holiness are inseparable.

Primordial Meditation uses a mantra chosen for us based on our birth information. It is usually a seed syllable that has a resonance with meaning when repeated. Deepak Chopra is an avid practitioner of this ancient practice of sound meditation in which you receive a personal mantra (or specific sound or vibration), which, when repeated silently, helps you to enter deeper levels of awareness.

The following is from *Meditation as Medicine* by Dharma Singh Khalsa, MD and is designed to influence the HPA axis (stress response initiator) to decrease the secretions of stress hormones. When doing the following chant, the midbrain, or limbic brain (the seat of our emotions as reviewed earlier on), along with the HPA axis, is relaxed. This, in turn, calms both the emotions and the stress response.

In an easy seated position or in a chair, relax hands on the knees. As you chant, visualize energy of the cosmos flowing in the top of your head and out your third eye point. The eyes are closed.

- Chant "Ong Namo Guru Dev Namo" three times. "I bow before my highest consciousness."
- Chant "Sa Ta Na Ma." Mudra: Sa, touch index to thumb; Ta, middle finger to thumb; Na, ring to thumb; Ma, pinky to thumb.
- Timing: Chant in normal voice for two minutes; whisper chant for two minutes; go deep within and chant silently for three minutes; whisper chant two minutes; normal voice two minutes. It should be eleven minutes total.
- Inhale deeply, exhale completely; lift spine and take several deep breaths.
- Birth, life, death, and rebirth are the meanings of Sa, Ta, Na, Ma; together they form Sat Nam—"my true identity." Focus on these concepts during the meditation.

Guided Meditation

For someone suffering with trauma, a guided meditation can be virtually risk-free. What I mean by that is that a person does not need to fear the perceived "wide open" space that meditation can create. Many with PTSD, anxiety, depression or other trauma symptoms will deeply fear silent meditation because thoughts, feelings and even memories can come up. I practice a guided meditation at least three times a week. It's the same one that I've been listening to for years.

Guided meditation (GM) involves you being guided through a journey by a leader, coach, teacher or practitioner. Guided meditation provides the road map of the journey so that you do not need to create it for yourself. It allows you to listen, absorb, and follow what is being said. GM helps disperse excess thought. I find it relaxing and a very "low maintenance" type of meditation, as you really don't need to do much of anything but listen and follow along. When I'm teaching my friends meditation, I will usually start with guided meditation. Visual components and somatic qualities are part of a GM journey. Guided meditation practices are very helpful for beginners as well as those with trauma symptoms. They are less intimidating and less distracting. Try different ones to see what works for you.

A note of caution: In 2003, I was teaching a YogaFit Level Three Training in Monterey, California. We teach basic meditation techniques in this workshop, so I decided to experiment with a guided meditation. I had just purchased a CD called "The Visit." In this meditation, the "guider" takes us on a journey that starts on the beach, goes into the forest, along a stream, and ends up a door. On the other side of the door, the "guider" tells us there is someone that has a message for us. "Each of them are waiting for you beyond the door." Needless to say, this did not go over well with everyone in the class. I jokingly say that I'm afraid this meditation may have caused some trauma. All humor aside, we need to be careful with the guided meditations that we chose for ourselves and others.

Sight—Visual Meditation

For many with trauma symptoms, closing the eyes can be scary. Keeping open eyes and watching something—a candle, the horizon, or even a bird—can truly help you maintain focus. Also, if you are a visual person, this may be a good style for you.

There are several different subsets of visual (open-eye) meditation:

Tratak involves fixing the eyes on something in the distance and not blinking. We spend all day looking at our cell phones or televisions or tablets—things close to our face—and this causes the muscles of our eyes to contract. Gazing into the distance allows those muscles to relax, restoring balance.

Palming the Eyes, while not technically a meditation practice, is an important adjunct practice for relaxing the musculature around the eyes and creating a situation more conducive to meditation and overall healing.

Yantra meditation focuses on sacred geometric shapes that correspond to different energetic qualities and archetypal energies. The shapes are often from the yoga tradition and represent different personified forces.

Mandalas are another type of sacred geometric design and are often complex codified designs from the Buddhist tradition. Pictures of labyrinths can be used for gazing as well.

Creating an Altar helps with visual meditation. Whether it is a candle or *yantra*, having a sacred object creates a meaningful focus. Even religious statues or deities can be used for visual meditation practice.

Somatic Meditation

The prefix *soma*-refers to the body, and somatic practices begin with an awareness of the body.

Often those who have experienced physical trauma in a way may shut down from their bodies or forget that they even have one. Somatic practices are a relatively safe way to reconnect without the movement of yoga *asana*. During somatic meditation, we get to feel and be in our bodies. We then may notice a part of our body and connect with body sensations of how our body feels. Somatic practices can also be moving practices. For many, running feels like a meditative event. Tai chi and other slow practices can also be moving meditations. Martial arts practices are more intense moving meditations. Swimming and surfing can also be meditative. Truly anything physical that engages the "flow state" (when you're completely in the zone and focused solely on the moment, action, and activity at hand) can be considered somatic.

Somatic meditation comes in three different forms and hits different senses.

- Eating is something we do multiple times a day and is a complete body experience. In order to make this into a meditative state, you need to fully appreciate the food are you eating. Take pause and be grateful. Breathe. Slow down and enjoy each piece of food you consume. Smell it. Chew slowly. Enjoy each bite. Be fully present in the physical experience.

- Using a counting tool (like a rosary, mala, or worry beads) or something to rub with the fingers gives you a tangible focal point. Beads can help count your mantras or breaths and allow you to be engaged with the hands and moment.

- Walking and feeling each step can be a profound form of meditation, engaging you into a flow state with the repetitive motion, which gains relaxation and insight.

Self-Healing Meditation

This meditation came to me in Tokyo as I was dealing with the carnage of a toxic situation that I allowed to infiltrate my being for far too long. It came spontaneously when I really needed it and my alternative coping skills (like exercise and yoga) were not an option due to my energy. I had no choice but to dive head first into my pain and the source of it. I am happy to say that to date I have no longer felt the depth of this pain. This self-healing meditation really worked for me and I hope it works for you too.

Set the intention that you will: clear and transmute all pain and blockages across all time, dimensions, space and reality.

If you are feeling pain, go into that pain fully and completely. For many that pain feels like a void, a dark hole. For me it felt like a dark well of pain, a funnel. Visualize your pain and fully immerse yourself in it. Imagine that black hole that is your pain, then watch yourself clean the walls, scrubbing them down. Spend time watching yourself physically doing the cleanup. Once that's done, fill that black hole, funnel, or tunnel up with a beautiful pink (or whatever bright color brings you joy) liquid, like a foam the consistency of a protein drink. Fill it to the top. Seal it up with a firmer substance, especially around the edges. I like to use the color orange.

Golden Brain Meditation

Sometimes when I meditate I like to send Golden Light to my brain. Golden Light is healing and repairing. Because I understand that my brain probably would have been able to function better had it not been for trauma, I often do this Golden Light meditation because I believe that it helps heal me.

I lie down and send energy in the color gold through my feet, up my body and into my brain. I amplify the color and light and imagine it weaving golden wires in my brain. I visualize it repairing and creating new neural pathways via that gold light. I watch it rebalance my brain.

Do this for about five to ten minutes per day.

Quick Tips to Practice Meditation

The following steps will help you establish a meditation practice:

1. Just do it. Commit to practicing your meditation for ten minutes (or more) each day. If that seems too overwhelming to you at the beginning, start with five minutes and tack on one minute every day. Set a timer and try to practice at the same time every day, which could be following your daily yoga practice. Find a comfortable place in your home (even if that means in the corner of your bedroom) and make that space a place of calm and love.

2. Choose a style for that day, don't be afraid to mix it up

3. Visualize an object or place in which you find peace, such as a quiet beach or your favorite flower.

4. Journal at the end of your practice so that you can keep track of your progress. For example, write down any techniques you tried and what you experienced practicing them. What were your thoughts and feelings before, during, and after meditating? Also, note if your practice revealed any solutions to questions or situations you've struggled to resolve. Finally, keep track of the benefits that you notice from incorporating meditation into your yoga practice.

Recognizing Your Success

How do you know if you are actually meditating successfully? For me, just the time and effort devoted to meditation is a success that means making the time and just showing up for it. Meditation is like a muscle, and we strengthen that muscle every time we use it. The meditative state is different for everyone. Some see stars, light, colors, while others see images, or connect to their angels or higher self. Others may see or feel nothing but pure space. Meditation gives me a wonderful state of "beingness," and deep sense of peace and calm. Just as there is no "right" version of a yoga pose, there is no "right" way to meditate.

As you begin to explore meditation and meditation techniques, remember that every day is different, every practice is different, and we are constantly faced with new struggles and challenges. Yet our inner truth remains the same; we need only to show up and practice.

Whatever your meditation practice, be sure to embrace the essence of YogaFit and let go of all judgment and expectation.

Survivor story: Marine

When I found YogaFit, I was desperate, addicted, wounded, closed off—disconnected. I was in my mid-thirties. I was suffering with severe posttraumatic stress symptoms related, in part, to a traumatic brain injury. I had been in the Marine Corps for sixteen years. I had been sexually abused for years as a child. My kid sister had been murdered in my early twenties. My wife had just left me. I attempted suicide.

When I survived, I wound up in military rehab treatment facility. While I was there, I had a psychiatrist who held my list of medications up in front of me and declared "this is not a sustainable life for you." He started to wean me off of the medications that were insulating me from my life. Under his care, he prescribed classes on mindfulness, writing, music therapy, and yoga. He suggested a different kind of yoga. This program had been designed by military yogis for the military. It was the Warrior Program.

This is where telling the story gets tricky. There is so much I want to say. I experienced so much in such a short amount of time. The Warrior Module is where I think I was first introduced to myself. I attended that module completely sold on the idea that I would never be able to sit quietly with my thoughts. Ever. I had been through too much. I was too broken. I was too unlovable. I had done and seen things that made me completely unredeemable. I believed that.

I learned that yoga is so much more than physical movement. I slowly started to learn about the connection between my mind and my body. I learned how to identify my feelings. I learned how to give them a name. I learned that they were almost always tied to stories that I told myself about other feelings. I learned about my samskaras. I learned that it was OK to set boundaries for myself.

In the beginning, I couldn't do yoga with the lights off. And that was OK! I needed to know that the doors were unlocked. And that was OK! The truth is, I didn't need any of those things. I just needed to be heard. I just needed to feel like my voice mattered. I had spent most of my life silencing myself. Yoga gave me the courage to hear the sound of my own voice and believe that it was good. I learned to make space where there was friction. Inside, outside, all around.

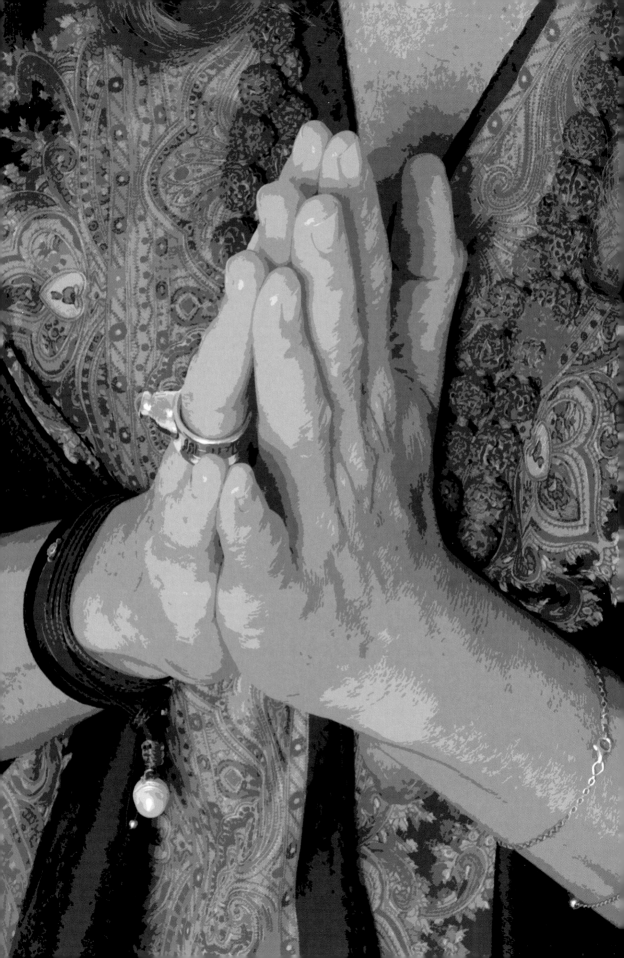

CHAPTER 7

Mantra, Music, and Sound Healing

"The processes that create sound into harmonious music are the same processes that govern all associating vibrations throughout the universe."

— FRITJOF CAPRA

About eight years ago, I went through a very difficult and traumatic experience. Fortunately, I had the tools of my yoga practice to rely on. I attended a Snatam Kaur concert in March of 2011. At this time in my life, I was on a strange autopilot, yet suffering at the core of my being. After the show, which was at the Wilshire Ebell Theatre, I purchased a few of her CDs. The one I put in my car's player was titled, *Mantra's for Precarious Times.* I could only play and listen to one song for three months. I love music—all types—but I simply could not listen to anything else. I was in so much pain. That mantra was Ra Ma Da Sa, and, as I later came to learn, it is the most healing of all chants and mantras.

This mantra evokes the sun, moon, earth, and Infinite Spirit in order to bring on healing. With eight sounds, it stimulates the central channels through the *kundalini* flow to activate healing. Apparently I am not the only one to have this experience; six months later, I was at Bhakti Yoga Shala in Santa Monica, California and it was very late at night. Jason Mraz and his guitar took the stage somewhere south of one a.m. He opened with the statement, "A year ago, I was on my bedroom floor in a very dark place. This chant came to me, and it saved my life." Then he did an acoustic version of Ra Ma Da Sa. To this day, I cannot listen to this chant without crying and going back to a very pivotal place on my spiritual journey. I released the album *YogaFit Presents Snatam Kaur* in 2012 so I could share her music with our network. I close every class with "By Thy Grace," and her music touches not only the heartstrings of my soul, but the very fibers of my being on many levels. Ra Ma Da Sa.

Mantras, chanting, and sound healing have literally saved my life. I use them on a daily basis to inspire, calm and clear the energy in my home and in myself. I also use these powerful teaching tools to create an experience for my students. Having had the blessing of teaching all around the world, I can say with confidence that music is not only universally transformative but individually, globally, and collectively healing.

Perhaps all of us have experienced that "one song" that we belted out as we were driving down the road or in the shower to help heal our heartbreak, or that one live performance where we felt the vibrations deep in our hearts and it became a part of us, a part of our story. Maybe you have an instrument that you play when you need solace, to escape.

Cultures around the world use sound and music extensively in diverse situations from celebrations to grieving, from war to peace, and as a part of their healing rituals. Why are sound and music so broadly used on the path to wellness? What makes them universal tools?

Sound and Music: A Primer

I'd like to thank YogaFit trainer Kristen Maybury—kirtan artist, sound therapist, E-RYT 500, C-IAYT—for contributing her wisdom to this section. Many researchers are now studying the power of sound, sound therapy, and music therapy as modalities of healing. For the sake of exploring sound and music as tools to process trauma, let's use the following terms and definitions.

- *Resonance* is the speed at which [the energy that makes up] any object (body part, brain) is vibrating. Everything has a healthy resonant frequency; that is a vibrational pattern requires the least amount of work to maintain—its natural state. And yes, in case you missed it, everything is vibrating.

- *Rhythm* is timing as it relates to sounds that are heard, biorhythms in the body, and lunar and solar cycles. When we catch ourselves using the phrases "we were just out of sync" or "that didn't resonate with me at all," those phrases are actually based in a deep understanding of the way we work (as vibrational beings).

- *Entrainment* happens when an object's frequency changes in response to a stronger frequency. Find the YouTube video of the numerous pendulums which when started out of sync, come into sync within a couple of minutes.

- *Coherence* describes the positive effects of entrainment. When we are exposed to particular sounds and or rhythms and are able to assimilate the healing frequencies on a vibratory level, healing occurs, and our unease is curtailed.

- *Dissonance* refers to the negative effects of entrainment. If the stronger frequency causes us to stray from a healing frequency and vibrate in a way that is not healthy, it becomes very difficult to break away from this new pattern and find our healthier frequency again.

- *Sound therapy* is a growing field where pure sound is used to elicit a particular reaction in a vibrating body (whole person or a specific body part). Tools in sound therapy can be as simple as a singing bowl or as complex as a cymatics machine.

- *Music therapy* uses organized, complex systems of sounds to elicit a particular reaction in a vibrating body. Many of us 'self-medicate' using songs from our youth or happy times in our lives, or songs where we identify with the lyrics. Formalized music therapy is systematic approach and often exposes the client to many different types and forms of music.

- *Mantra* is a Sanskrit word for "thinking tool" or "mind tool." Mantras from the yogic tradition are positive statements reflecting tantric views, such as different aspects of the divinity represented in each of us. To use a mantra, one repeats the phrase over and over (perhaps 108 times, which is an auspicious number from Vedic astrology) to get the most healing power from it.

What is the Yoga of Sound?

Nada Brahma (sound of the divine) was the first aspect of the practice of yoga to be described in the sacred yogic texts that have shaped yoga and kept it moving forward in time as a tool for transformation over the millennia.

"In the beginning was the word."Vibration started everything.

More than four thousand years ago, the *Rg* and *Sama Vedas* (two of the four ancient Vedic texts or hymns) dealt with recitation and chanting techniques, and yogis learned"Om"and the"Gayatri Mantra,"a prayer in song, those lines. Long before anything was written about where to safely keep your knees in Warrior One or how to use your core to lift into headstand, the buzz on the street was how to chant. Why? The "Gayatri Mantra"is so powerful because it invokes life. It does not invoke any deity, only the primordial and scared light of the divine itself. As it relates to trauma, light is an important element because of its power over darkness. My favorite chant from the "Gayatri Mantra" is from artist Deva Premal. In fact, I liked it so much, I doubled up on the tracks on YogaFit's Deva Premal Album.The "Gayatri Mantra" is considered the essence of hte Vedas.

Other yogic texts also discuss the power of sound as a tool of equanimity. The Nada Bindu Upanishad describes in great detail the liberation (mukta) one can experience by concentrating on a pure sound until even the sound itself is dissolved into the source. Then one attains the'true state' unaffected by anything from this world. In Patanjali's Yoga Sutras, he reminds the reader that yoga is quieting the mind and heart. He lists ceaseless chanting of mantra as one of the paths to the eighth limb of yoga, Samadhi, where there is no suffering. Patanjali also says that"Om"is God's name as well as form. Sound is consistently offered up as a tool of the practice throughout the development of the yoga tradition, which was, by the way, an oral tradition. All of these texts were chanted in their entirety, handed down from teacher to student, so that they could be deeply known—in the way you know something when you have internalized it to the point that it is a part of you—long before they were finally written down.

How Can Sound Help Us Heal From Trauma?

It's not only what sound and music do, but what they undo. When we allow ourselves to connect with the vibratory nature of sound and music, the judgment-related information processing in the discriminating mind turns off and our focus shifts to that of the experiential. Presence. Feeling. The more we learn about the brain, the more we know that experience is key to healing. Movement and flow are key to getting and keeping our energetic pathways clear. Just like the Essence of YogaFit (breathing, feeling, listening to the body; letting go of judgment, expectations, and competition; and staying in the present moment), the use of sound, music, and mantra shifts our focus to what is real, what is here, what is now, and how we can affect real change in our current state, personally, in our community, and globally.

Vibration opens the energetic pathways where *prana* flows. Thus, when we directly experience the healing vibration of sound, energy blocks can be removed, and healing and growth happen.

So where does the healing vibration come from?

Gloria Estefan may have been right when she sang "The Words Get in the Way." It's not the words *per se* (unless your words are in Sanskrit); it's the vibrational energy that holds the healing power. Let's remove the words from your favorite piece of music for now. What's left? Turns out there's a lot! Tone, pitch, timbre, rhythm, melody, harmony—each of these components of sound (and more complex, organized sounds as music) can have dramatic effects on our brain-wave state and our emotional state (or in yogic terms, our *citta vritti*), and therefore all aspects of our health—including the physical, emotional, mental, and spiritual—can benefit. Often song lyrics can carry extra layers of association which really do get in the way of letting go or quieting the mind.

Goldman (2002) writes that the secret healing sauce is the harmonics! The science to support that requires a bit of study, but the truth is that any sound that you hear is made up of an infinite number of sounds including the tone or pitch that your ears hear and many other tones above and below that one. The human ear is only capable of hearing between 20 and 20,000 Hz. Your best four-legged friend can hear more harmonics than you, which may explain how they can tell what kind of mood you're in and anticipate when you need love. Goldman also discusses how important it is to have space between the sounds for us to fully integrate the healing potential. Imagine music notes washing over you and each one already knows exactly where to land, in order to bring that part of you back in coherence. Health. Peace. Happiness. We must give it a moment to soak in and do its job before we bombard ourselves with the next stimulus. This is why, when we chant mantra, we leave a few moments of silence when the chant is complete.

At the YogaFit Mind-Body Fitness Conference's community *kirtan*, we share very special moments of shared vibration. When singing your favorite mantras together with a couple hundred of your fellow yogis, you get lost in the sounds around you, within you—you become the sound. Many students say it is one of their favorite memories from their teacher training because, for those brief moments, you're able to tap into the source and welcome in the healing vibrations that are stronger than the ebb and flow of the craziness of everyday life, and you are healed. You are restored. You are whole, and—if only for those fleeting moments—nothing else matters.

Incorporating Sound and Mantra into your Practice

Do you want to use sound therapy but are not sure where to start or how to do it?

Yogis who want to explore sound, mantra, and chanting often ask,"Do I have to be able to sing?""What song should I pick?""Can I just listen?""Which frequency crystal bowl should I buy?"

There is good news. Goldman (2002) suggests that: Frequency + Intention = Healing

So, even if we're not sure of the exact frequency to use, if our singing voice isn't perfect, if we play the wrong note, as long as our intention is pure and reflects a higher purpose of releasing trauma and freeing our mind and heart, healing will still occur. This simple formula beautifully opens up so many doors to healing. Letting go of expectations about what we"should" or"shouldn't" feel in any chakra or layer of self when we chant a particular mantra or listen to a particular piece of music is very liberating. We simply experience the sound and it is either healing and we continue, or it's not healing and we change what we expose ourselves to.

Do you need to learn Sanskrit?

Well, Sanskrit is the Language of Yoga—the original language of the sacred texts that defined and shaped the discipline of yoga—the *Vedas*, *Upanishads*, *Mahabharata*, *Ramayana*, *Yoga Sutras*, etc. It is an intrinsic language; the sound and the meaning are one. Some Sanskrit words just don't really translate. The vibration of the pronunciation is the meaning. This is strikingly evident when the Sri Yantra is produced by toning Om onto a tonoscope! If Om is God's name as well as form, then he's a tetrahedron inside concentric circles. I listen to Sanskrit chants often and, while I don't understand logically what they are saying, I believe that I do energetically.

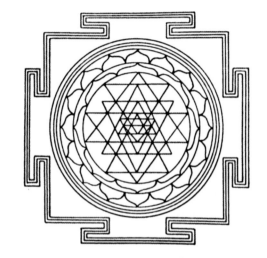

Carrying that 'intrinsic' idea one step further, David Frawley (2010) identifies the part of the body that is entrained by the vibrational energy surrounding different Sanskrit sounds. It really is a *deva lingua* (divine language).

You can learn more about the language of Sanskrit and feel the beautiful flow of pronouncing *Om namah shivaya*, or simply trust in the power of the vibration and welcome its healing energy into your being as the mantra washes over you as I do. Some may find it helpful to know the translation of the mantra before they listen to it over and over again. In that case, look it up and say a word of gratitude for the yogis over the millennia who not only passed down the oral tradition, but took the time to write these mantras down. Then a few of them even attempted to translate this beautiful vibrational language into our own. Others find a mantra uncannily comforting and healing without knowing how it translates on an intellectual level. They understand that the parts of you that need to know what it means, already do. They have recognized the vibrations as coherent and are already entraining towards without words and translations.

Passive versus Active Use of Sound and Music for Trauma

There are times for both, as there are very powerful benefits from receiving sound. Incredible healing energy can come from making sound as well. Let's examine a few ways to explore each approach and let's also create space and silence between the sounds where you can listen and feel, because feeling is what it's all about.

Receiving Sound

- YogaFit produces many downloadable albums, along with my meditations, which are available on iTunes.
- YouTube has great variations of the *Bhagavad Gita* in Sanskrit that I use daily.
- If you like the idea of listening to mantras performed in different ways to find one that resonates with you, check out New World Kirtan, a podcast. You can listen to all of the amazing *kirtan* artists chanting mantra in the beautiful playlists, then go to the website to see who they were and support them by purchasing their music.
- If you find a mantra that you like, type it into iTunes or Spotify and find different versions.
- Find a sound therapist in your area and book a Sound Bath. Your therapist will use singing bowls, drums, and other instruments to create an individualized 'bath' to wash away all energy blocks and get you on the path to healing.
- Listen to sounds in nature—your cat's purr, your dog's snore, a peaceful stream, singing birds—whatever is pleasing to you.

Making Sound

Your voice is the most powerful instrument in the world to bring healing into your mind, body, spirit because it is already perfectly coherent. It is already "tuned" to the best station. It is a shortcut to your very essence. Why is there so much resistance to vocalizing fear? Once you surpass that fear, magic happens. Your voice is your vibration and, according to the aforementioned formula, when your intention is from-the-heart pure, seeking healing, your voice literally cannot go wrong, so just sing! I often walk with one earbud in and sing—this way I can hear my voice and the music.

- Sing along to your favorite mantras. Use a mantra to ensure that you're singing inspirational vibrations (what happens to be on the radio may not contain the same energy). If you mispronounce the Sanskrit, just make a joyful noise. Some days, you just make a noise until it becomes joyful.

- Tone a vowel sound or *bija* mantra like Om, and pause. Listen and feel your response to that sound in the silence.

- Get a drum or a singing bowl. Yes, all instruments have particular ways they are played. These two general classes of instruments can be fairly easy to begin with. Set the intention for healing, then find a vibration that entrains you. Lose yourself in the rhythm and vibration while they clear away the blocks. I play music or chants for almost every occasion and I ask the universe to guide me to what type of music I need that day. It is no more unusual to hear Sanskrit chants than it is to hear rap, hip-hop, club music, or classical.

References
. . . .

Mantra Yoga and Primal Sound. 2010. David Frawley

Music as Yoga. 1956. Swami Sivananda

Healing Sounds. 2002. Jonathan Goldman

Your Brain on Music. Daniel Levitin

Sound Healing. Marjorie DeMuynck

Sacred Sounds. Ted Andrews

Music and Mantras. Girish

Survivor story: Rebecca

My story goes back to childhood (perhaps to conception!) and continues through adulthood. Sometimes days are challenging and do not feel quite successful, but I am thankful that I have yoga and Ayurveda to help manage choices that serve my health.

I am an identical twin. We share the same DNA. From conception I was/we were split in half—divided if you will. This created judgment, expectations, and competition right from the start. Our parents divorced when we were very young—another separation. I believe that I crave yoga, which means union in Sanskrit, so much because I am seeking union within myself and those around me. Most of my life, I dealt with worry and fear in some way or another. At the age of fourteen, I was sexually abused. I kept it a secret for years, and during that time, it was a struggle to develop healthy dating relations. At the age of nineteen, I decided to seek psychotherapy, which is when I was first introduced to yoga.

My first experience with yoga was *The Yoga Sutra of Patanjali*. It felt like I hit the jackpot because it was about how to control the mind. I used that book a lot to help with all of the irrational thoughts that I gave myself and those thoughts from other people's words that did not serve and support me in a positive way.

At the age of twenty, I was in an abusive relationship mentally, physically, and emotionally. The boyfriend had his own issues with grief, loss, drugs, and alcohol. One night, we were fighting and he put a gun to my head threatening to kill himself and me. Thankfully, I survived. Since that experience, I had to deal with body dysmorphic disorder, disordered eating, binge eating, and stressing out about being healthy with active running and even yoga. During my twenties and thirties, I worked in a pediatric office, and I remember always having a fear or worry about being pregnant and meeting the right person to have kids and a family with.

I was diagnosed with uterine cancer five years ago. I had three genetic tests come back inconclusive. My oncologists said it was bad luck. I always thought that was odd, being a firm believer in yoga and Ayurveda, holistic health, and mind-body connections. I was also introduced to the book by Deb Shapiro, *Your Body Speaks Your Mind* in YogaFit classes. It's a constant reference in my life and yoga teachings.

While studying Ayurveda two years ago, I found what I believe was the reason why I got cancer. I am a *Vata Kapha* type. Binge Eating Disorder is a *Vata Kapha* imbalance. What I learned in Ayurveda was that we (humans) potentially give ourselves our own diseases. Of course, I didn't know this prior to learning Ayurveda. Years ago, I created my own mindful eating plan through the eight limbs of Yoga focusing on the *yamas* and *niyamas* to help myself with my eating disorder, but what I learned through Ayurveda was that the first part of digestion is *prana* and a clear mind. I used to believe that the first stage of digestion was in the mouth, chewing—which is a big part of it, chewing slowly—but that saying "it's not what you're eating, it's what's eating you" is valid and holds a lot of value! One of my yoga teachers said something that I always remembered, "You can have the cleanest diet known to man, exercise every day, and practice yoga, but if you are not taking care of your thoughts, it is more detrimental to your health than eating a hamburger!" Ayurveda believes in the six-taste theory and the seven tissues in the body. The reproductive organs are the seventh tissue (the last to get "fed"). I believe that I wasn't feeding myself well enough for my tissues to be fed efficiently, and I wasn't feeding my soul enough love either.

I have obsessive compulsive disorder (OCD), general anxiety, an eating disorder (binge), slight depression at times, PTSD from trauma of abuse, and cancer.

I have always used yoga and Ayurveda (since I was in my early twenties) to help find balance in my life with all things, but having cancer helped me find freedom from stress—even stressing about being healthy! Now I focus on being happy and loving myself. I use the YogaFit essence (letting go of competition, expectations, judgement) daily. At times my problems do not leave me completely, so I rely on the Ayurvedic principle, "Like increases like, and opposites cure."

When I am grieving, I turn it into gratitude.

When I am stressed, I breathe.

I use yoga poses and meditation (anything and everything that I can!) as a way to gain strength and flexibility in my body and to get back in touch with my body to help move energy.

When I am feeling unbalanced, I practice routine self-care regimens of Ayurveda. I use many of the *Dinacharya* acts to keep me on a balance to take care of and honor myself. I do the best that I can every day.

I would be extremely lost or dead, quite frankly, in one way or another without yoga and Ayurveda in my life.

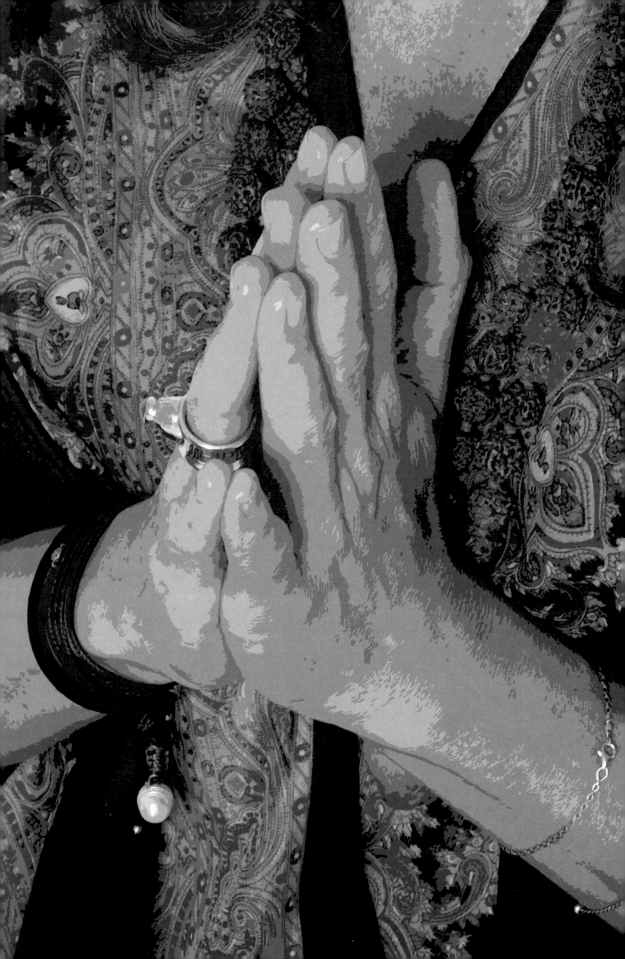

CHAPTER 8

Ayurvedic Hacks For Stress, Anxiety, and Depression

"Fulfill all your duties; action is better than inaction. Even to maintain your body, Arjuna, you are obliged to act."

—Bhagavad Gita 3:9

What is Ayurveda?

Ayurveda is a holistic system of health and wellness that is often described as being a complementary or sister science to yoga. "Science of Life" is the most frequently translated version of the Sanskrit name "Ayurveda." The teachings of Ayurveda offer a comprehensive system of lifestyle interventions to support physical, mental, emotional, and spiritual health, and are focused on the overall balance of the system. This is significant in addressing trauma. I use Ayurvedic "hacks" on a daily basis to help me calm my nervous system, enhance energy, stay balanced, detox when needed, and just feel generally better.

We will review a number of Ayurvedic hacks (or tools) that help build resilience and can even be significant in helping to repair the nervous system and the body as a whole.

The system of Ayurveda offers an understanding of our individuality through the identification of different body types. These categories can explain why people have different vulnerabilities and how they are affected by trauma, how dealing with trauma can affect people differently, and why different remedies work for different people.

Ayurveda and the Doshas

In Ayurveda, the doshas are identified as categories of energy. There are three doshas: vata, pitta, and kapha. Each one of us is made up of a combination of these in varying amounts. We may have a predominant dosha or doshas. According to Ayurveda, our health and well-being are affected by whether our individual combination of the doshas is in a state of balance or imbalance.

Most often, an excess of any of the doshic energies leads to greater imbalance. Balancing the dosha involves bringing in more of the opposite qualities.

The doshas relate to body types, and these include physical as well as psychological characteristics. The qualities of the different doshas can affect our resilience as well our responses to trauma and traumatic events.

Vata

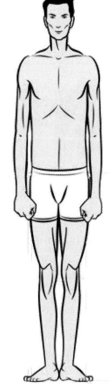

Physically, the category of the vata dosha is similar to what we would call an ectomorph. This shows up as being generally slender with naturally less body fat. The vata dosha is naturally cold. People with a predominance of the vata dosha can often have reduced resilience or the feeling of less of a buffer overall compared to the other categories. For this reason, techniques that help a person feel more grounded and more centered become important for building or maintaining balance.

The vata dosha is responsible for the workings of the nervous system and all movement in the body. Because the vata dosha is connected to the nervous system, the

Ectomorph

disturbances of one affect the other. Building our resilience and healing from the effects of trauma is related to balancing the activity of the vata dosha and properly caring for and feeding the nervous system.

● **Strengths:** The vata dosha is related to creativity, flexibility, expansive thoughts and ideas, intuition, new beginnings, and all movement.

● **Challenges:** Since the vata dosha is related to change, a lot of change or movement can increase or imbalance the vata dosha. This is especially the case when it comes to trauma, but also includes travel and even positive life events.

When vata is out of balance, some of the things we can experience include the following: hypersensitivity to stimulation, increased fear, anxiety, worry, forgetfulness, difficulty falling asleep or staying asleep, constipation, digestive disorders, hypersensitivity, depression, lack of focus and lack of clarity, excessively dry skin, loss of appetite, and feelings of not being grounded.

Excess stress can lead to either weight loss (from loss of appetite and digestive imbalances) or weight gain (from a person overeating as a means of feeling grounded or calming the nervous system).

● **How to Balance:** Some of the ways to balance the vata dosha include the following: favoring routine and regularity, such as eating meals at predictable times during the day; regular trauma-sensitive massage and self-massage techniques; eating warm, comforting, grounding foods; reducing use of stimulants, including coffee and other forms of caffeine, as well as refined sugars; increasing intake and use of healthy fats, such as omega-three fatty acids and foods like avocado; yogic practices that are grounding and calming; and listening to uplifting music.

Pitta

Physically, the pitta dosha is most often the mesomorph
body type, or the person in the middle, who has some
stamina and good muscle tone that benefits from
training. The pitta dosha is connected to our digestion
and metabolism, so someone with a predominance
of the pitta dosha may have a strong digestion, but
at the same time may be prone to hyperacidity,
ulcers, or other situations where the acidity of the
digestive system may be in excess. The pitta dosha is
naturally hot. The energy of the pitta dosha may have
challenges with anger when in excess. When it comes to
addressing trauma, holding onto anger or the presence
of underlying or unexpressed anger can be particular
concerns.

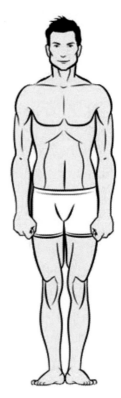

Mesomorph

● **Strengths:** The pitta dosha is related to digestion and metabolism, as well
as our focus, discipline, and passion in life. A naturally competitive nature is
part of this category, so channeling the competitive energy for positive effects
is important to maintain balance.

● **Challenges:** When in a state of imbalance, the pitta dosha can experience
anything related to hyperacidity in all systems of the body, as well as excess
anger and irritability. Other challenges related to an imbalance of pitta are
inflammation, irritable eyes, headaches, excess heat, and difficulty sleeping.
   Pitta-influenced patterns of weight gain can lead to weight gain around the
center of body. Excess of stress hormones can negatively impact abdominal
weight gain since the receptors in this area are sensitive to stress hormones.

● **How to Balance:** Anything that is cooling is soothing to the energy of
the pitta dosha. Foods, drinks, people, and practices. Water is a key remedy;
staying hydrated, swimming, bathing, taking showers, and even taking a walk
with a view of the water are practices to calm pitta. It's also important to
balance by making sure to take good care of digestion. Processing emotions

is a significant part of mental digestion and important for maintaining balance for the pitta dosha. Practices that help release pent-up energy, channel competitive energy in positive ways, reduce anger, and promote calm are balancing.

Kapha

People who have a predominance of the kapha dosha fall into the endomorph category when it comes to body type. There may be a tendency toward being more insulated and naturally having denser bone structure and more padding, as well as greater stamina and even the ability to build strength and develop endurance when properly trained. That being said, the kapha dosha needs to spend more time working out and might benefit from a personal trainer or attending classes for the support and encouragement. The stamina and insulation of the kapha dosha may make it seem like this category of dosha or person is immune to the effect of stress or trauma, but in actuality there may be an accumulation that builds to a person's breaking point.

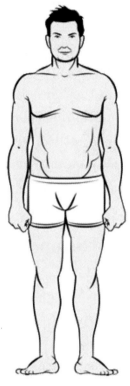

Endomorph

● **Strengths:** Endurance, endurance, endurance. This can be both a strength and a challenge, as the quality of endurance for the kapha dosha can mean endurance even in situations that a person is better off leaving. Besides endurance, the energy of the grounded and stable kapha dosha sets up good sleep and steadiness. The calm demeanor of this category can have a positive influence on other people as well. The energy of the kapha dosha is also the energy of unconditional love and nurturing.

● **Challenges:** Back to this endurance and holding on to the point of being stuck. The energy of kapha is not a fan of change, so making shifts, even positive ones, can sometimes be hard. When it comes to things being stuck, this can include weight gain as well as any kind of excess in life: stuff at home, ideas, grudges, and jealousies. Kapha dosha is prone to congestion of all kinds and tends to be cold and damp.

● **How to Balance:** This is the dosha that needs some stimulation, but it may need an approach that involves working up to things in stages. Think building conditioning rather than starting with a marathon on day one. The naturally cold energy needs to be warmed, and the dampness needs to be dried. Sitting in a sauna can be stimulating, but if someone is overweight, limit the time so as not to overwhelm circulation. Regular exercise and conditioning is important. In terms of food, smaller portions, use of spices for warmth and stimulation, and lots of vegetables are supportive. Since emotions are often held in or even suppressed, fully processing emotional states is vital.

The Support of Lifestyle Medicine

In the field of lifestyle medicine, Ayurveda takes the approach that everything has the potential to contribute to our path and practice of healing and wholeness. Lifestyle interventions are an integral part of this approach. This is not to say that lifestyle alone will necessarily be enough to even reverse the effects of persistent trauma. Yet in the teachings of Ayurveda, daily routine and lifestyle practices can support the efficacy of everything else that a person is doing to address the effects of trauma on mind, body, and spirit.

There is a long history of this use of traditional medicine. The efficacy of these practices are a robust area of current research, including in PTSD and persistent trauma.

Ayurveda offers a wide range of suggestions for implementing supportive habits. We could think of them as modern hacks for happiness. Ayurveda has a long list of tips for calming the nervous system, building our resilience and resistance, and generally upgrading our body, mind, and spirit. We can use these practices along with yoga to manage stress and the physiological effects of trauma.

Begin with Compassion

Any practice of transformation begins with an acknowledgment and acceptance of where you are now. Infuse your daily routine with self-compassion.

Compassion Hack:Throughout your day, recognize self-critical thoughts. Repeat compassionate self-talk.

According to Ayurveda, infusing compassion in a healing journey is a key ingredient for success. A 2019 study published in *Behaviour Research and Therapy* confirms this. The authors say that self-compassion is even a predictor of PTSD recovery.

The Importance of Experimentation

Give yourself permission to process! Experiment with ideas and awareness to discover what works for you. Know that not every type of practice and intervention works for everyone.

Since Ayurveda is based on the premise that we each experience the effects of the doshas differently, different interventions and techniques will work for us. We have different needs for balance and for emotional, physical, and even spiritual regulation. Discovering the helpful hacks for our own unique nature come from experimentation.

Add instead of Subtract

When we begin considering our lifestyle, we may start to think we have to give up all of the habits we love. We might start naming our indulgences and vices. From the perspective of Ayurveda, start thinking about what you can add to your life. Before you panic about your lack of time, this isn't about adding a lot of tasks to your day—just adding a bit more intentional support to your regimen. People tend to find that by adding in a bit more support here and there, some of the less supportive habits may start to drop away.

Cultivating Calm

The nervous system is an important modulator of our experience. Ayurvedic practices can help calm the nervous system, which then has global effects on our well-being. These include everything not only in this chapter, but throughout this book.

Ayurvedic Hacks for Getting Grounded

The phenomenon of being grounded involves being centered, focused, embodied, and in better control of all of your faculties. It is a helpful state of being for reducing anxiety, dealing with depression, and addressing trauma.

Walk in the Grass in Bare Feet

What it is: Take off your shoes and allow the soles of your feet to come in contact with the sand, grass, rocks, or soil.

Why it works: People who talk about the phenomenon of earthing describe the electron transfer between living systems and the electromagnetic field of the earth. That may sound a bit esoteric, but research does confirm the antioxidant effects of walking barefoot on the earth. Some of the additional benefits include stimulation of reflexology points on the feet as well as articulation of the joints of the foot and the benefits of the massaging action of walking barefoot on the fascia and other tissues of the feet.

Forest Bathing

What it is: The Japanese name for this practice is Shinrin-Yoku. Distinct from hiking, forest bathing is the practice of simply spending time in nature without any agenda. You can be in a remote area or even a park or urban forest to experience the benefits. Find a spot you love that is easy to access and just go outside. Refrain from text messaging.

Why it works: Proven stress relief comes from spending unstructured time in nature. There is a growing body of research that confirms the benefits, which include: stress reduction, improved immune system function, and a reduction in anxiety and depression.

Gardening

What it is: Just like it sounds, gardening (called horticultural therapy) has benefits in addition to eating the fresh tomatoes you have grown.

Why it works: Gardening is shown to reduce depression, uplift mood, and improve memory. Some of this may be related to the effects of being outside in the sunshine and fresh air, as well as enjoying the benefits of moving and getting exercise. There is also a body of research that reveals that being exposed to soil microbes actually has a similar effect on the brain and nervous system as some anti-depressants.

Begin with the Breath to Calm the Nervous System

Throughout this book, you've been reading about how the breath is important for healing the effects of trauma. Remember that our breath is a constant companion for us throughout our day. The time we spend on the yoga mat or the meditation cushion provide us with the practice that allows us to bring our attention to our breath in stressful moments. Examples of this can be everything from driving in the car, flying, giving a presentation at—or just going to—work, taking an exam, or—well—just about everything. Make it a practice to simply pause and take a deep breath. Make it a habit to slow down the pace of your breath whenever you can. Think of it as an instantaneous attitude adjustment.

Ayurvedic Hacks to Improve Digestion

Health in the body begins with digestion. According to Ayurveda, we're not only what we eat, we are what we digest. How well we digest our food sets us up for how well we are able to absorb the building blocks of everything from the neurotransmitters that manage our mood, to the hormones that control our homeostasis, to the tissue of our bones and muscles that literally support us. Keep reading the chapters here for suggestions for supportive eating and nutrition.

When You're Eating, Eat.

We love multitasking, but bringing our attention and awareness to our food helps us enjoy more efficient digestion. Paying attention to our food really does make a difference. Also, when you're reading or watching something while you're eating, you're also eating that too. Think about it...do you really want to eat today's news or yesterday's gossip? When you pay attention to your food, you may even slow down and feel more satisfied.

Why it works: Mindful eating or what is also called attentive eating helps with weight control as well as stress reduction. Eating mindfully is also an important remedy for addressing the negative effects of trauma.

Hot Water with Lemon.

Start out your day with some hot water with lemon or sip on it throughout the day. I do this every single morning, along with an affirmation or intention before drinking it. This classic Ayurvedic recommendation is simple yet effective. You don't have to give up your coffee or your favorite morning beverage, just add this to your morning.

Why it works: Beginning your day with a bit of clarity has powerful detoxifying effect. When we encourage detoxification, even just a little bit, we can help release anything we may be holding onto. This can include physical metabolic waste as well as any mental clutter.

Leave Time Between Meals

Allow yourself time to digest one meal before eating the next one. Depending on your own metabolism, you may be eating a few small meals with snacks or you may just be eating meals. Either way, give yourself some time and space between sitting down to eat and pay attention to your food as you eat it.

Digestive Teas

Drinking herbal tea, such as ginger, peppermint, lavender, tulsi, turmeric, or cinnamon can help stimulate digestion, improve detoxification, and strengthen the immune system.

Triphala

The herbal blend triphala is a remedy used in Ayurveda for overall detoxification. Some people find that it may have the effect of improving elimination and maintaining regularity, although it is not a laxative. I use triphala at least once a month. Ladies, it's great to use just before your menstrual cycle starts to eliminate excess bloating.

Triphala is a mixture of three dried and powdered fruits: amalaki (Indian gooseberry, or *Phyllanthus emblica*), haritaki (myrobalan or *Terminalia chebula*), and bibhitaki (*Terminalia bellirica*). They have the effect of balancing all three doshas and nurturing the tissues of the body while, at the same time, encouraging detoxification.

This is best taken away from meals, rather than with meals.

How to Use it: Capsules or tablets, tea (one-fourth to one-half teaspoon with a cup of water), cold infusion (one-half teaspoon in water, stir, let sit overnight, drink the liquid in the morning).

Why it works: According to Ayurveda, since triphala can balance all three doshas, it has supportive effects on healing. As trauma can affect accumulation in the body, triphala is also supportive as it helps to reduce accumulation.

Bathroom Hack: Tongue Scraping

Keep a tongue scraper next to your toothbrush for a three-minute detox when you're completing your oral hygiene. I've been using tongue scrapers for over twenty years—every time I brush my teeth I scrape. I bought my first one in the Indian markets in Singapore where I was doing a YogaFit training in 1999. Tongue scrapers are an inexpensive, easy-to-clean, long-lasting tool for detoxification. A 2018 study in *Clinical Oral Investigations* demonstrated that tongue scraping reduces inflammatory markers and improves breath and other hygiene parameters.

What to look for: Metal tongue scrapers are more effective, easier to clean, and last longer than plastic scrapers. You can find stainless steel, plastic, or even silver tongue cleaners in a variety of places.

How to use: Either before or after brushing your teeth and flossing, look in the mirror, and stick out your tongue. Place the tongue scraper on the back of your tongue and gently scrape forward. Spit and rinse. Repeat as desired. Clean the scraper after each use.

Why it works: The effects of trauma, depression, and anxiety can affect hygiene, including oral care. Tongue scraping improves oral hygiene, which can also improve self-esteem. Tongue scraping reduces inflammation, which also has an impact on immunity.

A 2018 systematic review published in the *Journal of Inflammation Research* identified evidence that there is relationship between PTSD and a chronic low-grade inflammatory state. This is significant as there is wide-ranging discussion in medical and scientific research about the connection between persistent inflammation and a wide range of chronic diseases. Many Ayurvedic remedies are powerful and effective because they serve to reduce inflammation.

Turmeric as an Anti-inflammatory

The spice turmeric is related to ginger and has a long history of use in Ayurveda because it reduces inflammation. It has received attention in modern scientific research for this effect.

Turmeric is best taken with food, and having turmeric with some form of fat helps increase the absorption of the active curcuminoids. There are studies that show that black pepper can increase the bioavailability of some of the compounds in turmeric, but turmeric is effective even if taken without black pepper.

Add turmeric to food and recipes, try taking capsules or other supplements, slice the fresh root and boil it for tea, or make golden milk.

GOLDEN MILK

For one cup of milk, use one-half teaspoon of powdered turmeric.

Add additional spices as desired: pinch of black pepper, one-fourth teaspoon of grated ginger or small piece of sliced ginger, cardamom, nutmeg, cinnamon, or vanilla.

If not using full fat milk, add a healthy oil like coconut to improve absorption of turmeric.

On the stove, mix the milk with the spices. Warm and stir. Add honey after heating if desired.

Why it works: This warm and spicy drink has anti-inflammatory effects and can also be calming for the nervous system. Warm milk can help improve sleep.

Tulsi (Holy Basil or Indian Basil)

Tulsi or holy basil (*Ocimum sanctum*) is an adaptogen, which means it supports numerous systems in the body. It has stress relieving and anti-inflammatory effects. The adaptogens are a class of herbs that have strengthening and tonic effects on the entire system, including the endocrine or hormonal systems, the nervous system, and the immune system. They are often called adaptogens because they help the body adapt to stressful situations. The tonic effects of these herbs can be supportive for addressing the effects of trauma.

Some adaptogens that are becoming more commonly used include: reishi and chaga mushrooms, goji berries, maca, rhodiola, ashwagandha, astragalus, gotu kola, bacopa monnieri, ginseng (Siberian ginseng and panax ginseng), and tulsi.

How to use it: Drink tulsi tea.

Why it works: Naturally caffeine-free, this uplifting tea has anti-inflammatory, stress-relieving, anxiety-relieving, and depression-reducing properties. Drink hot or cold throughout the day. Different blends offer a variety of flavors.

Ginger

Ginger, like turmeric, has a variety of well-researched anti-inflammatory effects. In addition, ginger helps regulate the immune system and can stimulate digestion. PTSD and other trauma-related syndromes can negatively affect digestion.

How to use it: Drink ginger tea or cook with ginger.

Why it works: Ginger has supportive systemic effects on digestion, the immune system, and inflammation. It tastes good and has overall uplifting effects, according to Ayurveda.

Chyawanprash

This Ayurvedic food is a jam that is made from the antioxidant-rich fruit amla or amalaki, with a number of other added medicinal herbs and culinary spices. You can eat it any time of day by the spoonful, on toast, over breakfast cereal, or with tea or milk for an energizing boost.

There are a variety of brands and variations of this traditional recipe.

Why it works: The nourishing herbs in chyawanprash are tonics for the immune system, strengthen the body overall, provide stress resilience, and can even uplift mood.

Smoothies for recovery: If you're a smoothie person, fine-tune your blends to support healing. Reduce added sugars and add in adaptogenic herbs and healthy fats. Try infusing your blends with vitamin and mineral-rich greens.

The Magic of Music

Dancing, even just putting on a tune and dancing in your living room, can lift your spirits. Taking a dance break during the day can be a cheap and easy remedy on your healing journey.

Why it works: Research confirms the benefits of dancing, from improving memory to uplifting mood. In moments when you need a quick attitude adjustment, shut the door, put on a song you love, dance it out, and ride the endorphins. Dancing and yoga are my favorite forms of movement.

Ayurvedic Sleep Strategies

Daily sleep is an important part of the body's repair mechanism. During stages of deep sleep, our bodies produce the human growth hormone and other factors necessary for repair. In addition, dreaming is an important part of our psychological process and capacity for healing. It is known that all forms of trauma can disrupt our sleep patterns.

Follow sleep hygiene recommendations. These include making sure to stop drinking caffeine in a timely fashion before going to bed. You may even want to cut out the caffeine after noon or two p.m. if you have trouble sleeping. Some studies suggest that even though you may fall asleep after ingesting caffeine, it may affect your ability to enter into stages of deep sleep. Try blackout curtains. Remove electronics and lights from your bedroom. Use sleep mode on electronics to dim lights if you do use them, but it's recommended to give yourself space between screen-time and sleep.

Self-Massage for Self-Care

Foot Massage before Bed

What it is: One of the top Ayurvedic practices is to massage the feet at night while in bed. Using some easily absorbed oil heightens the benefits. Massaging the feet calms the vata dosha, reduces stress and anxiety, and promotes sounds sleep. I do this at least once a week, more if I am traveling often—my feet will actually tell me when they need it.

Why it works: Part of the benefit comes from stimulating the reflexology points on the feet. In addition, foot massage calms the nervous system. Some Ayurveda-recommended oils for foot massage include: Shea butter, sesame oil, coconut oil, almond oil, and jojoba oil. Personally, I like to use thick castor oil or coconut oil. Make sure you put on thick socks after you apply the oil. They should be very absorbent but thick enough so you don't get oil on your sheets or slip on the floor when you get up. I use ankle high thick grey cotton socks so I can oil my feet and ankles thoroughly.

Oil Your Scalp or Massage Your Head

We know the positive effects of a head or scalp massage on relaxation. Try giving yourself a scalp massage, or rub a little bit of oil into the scalp before bed.

Why it works: Just as we have an abundance of pressure points on the feet, we have a number of pressure points around the head and scalp. Oiling the scalp can also be calming to the vata dosha. Do this an hour before you shampoo or, if you can, before you go to sleep.

Foods that Support Sleep

Reducing refined sugars, especially before bed, is helpful as refined sugars have a stimulating quality. Foods like warm milk, chickpeas, dates, coconut, and coconut oil can be helpful for calming the nervous system to support sound sleep.

In Ayurveda, Abhyanga Is the Practice of Using Oil for Massage

Why it works: Massage stimulates the release of hormones and neurotransmitters that are calming to the nervous system, such as oxytocin and serotonin. Massage also encourages self-compassion and self-acceptance. Whether doing self-massage or getting a massage, there is also a benefit from strengthening the buffer or barrier between you and the outside world, which can improve resilience and reduce hypersensitivity.

Getting a Massage

Choose a trauma-sensitive massage therapist who you feel comfortable working with. It can be helpful to talk about your specific concerns and needs before or at the beginning of your session. Massage can be confrontational or be a trigger when addressing trauma, so sensitive professional help is important.

When you don't have time to visit a foot reflexologist or massage therapists, you can work these points yourself. Keep a ball or a set of balls under your desk or in your living room to have at the ready for stress relief. Why it works: Many traditional systems of healing recognize the presence of pressure points on the feet that correspond with other areas of the body. Releasing tension and stimulating the pressure points on the feet have powerful systemic effects. Research studies in pain management describe how foot massage can be helpful for relieving pain in a variety of situations.

Use of Oils for the Nervous System

Many Ayurvedic hacks use various forms of oil to support the activity of the nervous system. This includes on the body and in food. Choose easy-to-digest, healthy, raw oils. For food, try avocado, coconut oil, ghee, nuts, and nut butters, as well as vegetable oils such as olive, grapeseed, almond, walnut, and others.

Why it works: Oils are grounding and soothing. They nourish the skin and the tissues. Oils provide food for the nervous system, build the buffers of the body, and provide the building blocks for many neurotransmitters and hormones. I add generous amounts of flax seed oils into my daily protein drinks—it makes a big difference in my mood and balance and is great for the skin.

Nasya—Nose Oil

What it is: Nasya or nose oil, is an Ayurvedic self-care practice in which a mix of vegetable-based oils, sometimes ghee, herbal infused oils, and essential oils are placed in the nose. You tilt the head back and place three to five drops in one nostril, breath in deeply, and allow the oils to coat the inside of the nostrils. I use nose oils almost daily and multiple times while flying on an airplane to keep the nasal passages lubricated and the germs out.

Why it works: There is a close relationship between the olfactory system (which senses smell) and the emotion and memory-modulating limbic system. In Ayurveda, the use of smell and the use of oils are hacks that help balance the activity of the nervous system. Also, a bit of oil in the nostrils is calming to the vata dosha and can help reduce anxiety and depression. You can find nose oils readily available.

Aromatherapy, Ayurveda, and Addressing Trauma

Since smell is so closely connected to our emotional state and our memory, we can use aromatherapy as a therapeutic intervention any time of the day.

Why it works: Aromatherapy is an immediate attitude adjustment that affects the limbic system of the brain, a set of regions that regulate fear, anxiety, memory, and other processes. In Ayurveda, aromatherapy is valued for its easy-to-use positive benefits, without side effects.

Ways to use aromatherapy:

- Set up a diffuser in your home. I have two going at all times: one by the front door to greet my guests and myself when I come home, and one in my bedroom.
- Spray scents on your pillow to encourage sleep.
- Add a couple of drops of essential oils to the soles of your feet for immediate absorption and to calm the nervous system.
- I like to put peppermint in and behind my ears before a workout. I also put Breathe oil blend from dōTerra under my nose before an outdoor walk or workout.
- Use a roller ball of aromatherapy oils on the inside of the wrists, the neck, or around the chest. I use Whisper oil blend by dōTerra or straight-up sandalwood.
- Place a few drops on a cotton ball to have beside you on your yoga mat or to smell during meditation. Tuck it inside your clothing.
- Spray your yoga mat with diluted essential oils. Just make sure you don't slip!

Doshic Effects of Aromatherapy

In general, grounding, earthy scents are calming to the vata dosha: vetiver, sandalwood, patchouli, nag champa, frankincense, and palo santo.

Sweet and cooling scents are calming to the pitta dosha: rose, jasmine, peppermint, and lavender.

Uplifting and stimulating scents are balancing to the kapha dosha: rosemary, citrus, and cinnamon.

I use eucalyptus in the mornings, lavender and patchouli at night, and spray my bedding down daily.

I also like to keep a spray bottle with essential oils added to a facial toner in my fridge and spray my face a few times a day. Just make sure you keep your eyes closed until the oil settles and keep the spray away from your eyes.

Keep Practicing

Try incorporating healing hacks from Ayurveda throughout your day and integrate them into your routine. Journal the effects and benefits you experience and keep experimenting to discover the practices that work for you. Remember to incorporate self-compassion and kind thoughts to strengthen the positive benefits of your supportive daily routine.

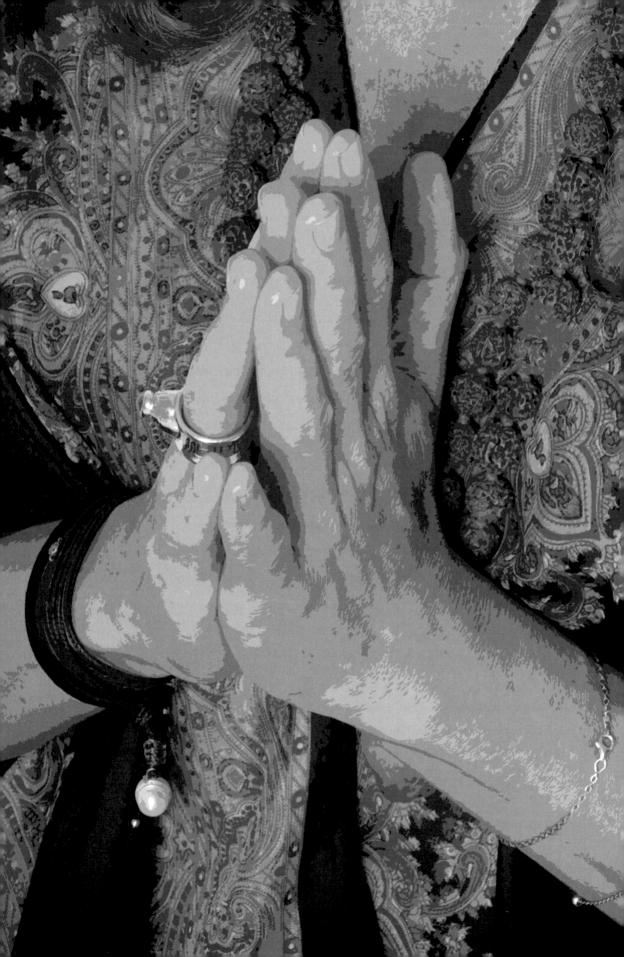

CHAPTER 9

Clean Eating and Managing Your Moods

"One can have no success at yoga if one eats too much or eats too little. But if you are moderate in eating, playing, sleeping, staying awake, and avoiding extremes in everything you do, you will see that yoga practices eliminate your pain and suffering."

—BHAGAVAD GITA 6:16–17

"Those of tranquil temperament prefer foods that increase vitality, longevity, and strength; foods that enhance physical health and make the mind pure and cheerful; foods with substance and natural flavor; foods that are fresh, with natural oils and agreeable to the body."

—BHAGAVAD GITA 17:8

We are what we eat. Food affects mood, and what we consume each day plays a vital role in our overall mental and physical health. Making healthier choices will help lift our moods, keep us in proper weight for our unique bodies, and provide a long-lasting support in energy.

Self-care is critical for anyone dealing with trauma. The foods that we eat can both enhance and support our healing, or get in the way of the healing to occur. While dealing with trauma, it can be difficult to eat well, stand up and go to the grocery store, let alone meal prep. However, proactive self-care is one of the primary aspects in gaining back strength and staying in the present.

We've touched on how many trauma survivors can easily slip into addiction as a way of self-medicating—food addiction is perhaps one of the most pervasive addictions that exist. For many, to rely on food to soothe and comfort is more socially acceptable than becoming an alcoholic or drug addict. Food is a lot more readily available because we *need* to eat, so people can easily slip into food addiction and derail a healthy body.

In a nation where more than 40 percent of the population is obese and 66 percent are overweight, clearly there is a lot of work to do here. New studies show that, after briefly leveling off, the US obesity rates are climbing again, and researchers have found that the leveling-off trend may have been short-lived. As stated in my book *YogaLean*, I believe that, for most people, being overweight, and particularly obese, is not unlike a hoarding disorder. After all, what is excess weight? More weight than your body needs to carry, and a result of ingesting more food than you need.

It's also important to note that body image can affect your mood. If you struggle through trauma and begin to notice a decline in your eating habits, it may also be reflected in your body image. Yoga and the practices that go along with it, help gain perspective back and develop a stronger relationship with how you view and feel in your physical body. Every time you step onto the mat, you are asked to feel. Your body is there to help you, and it's important to ensure you are helping it.

Body Mass Index (BMI) is one way to measure and define Adult Overweight and Obesity. A high BMI can be an indicator of high body fat. I find the ranges of what is "normal body weight" to be too large, and they certainly do not take into account things like body type—ectomorph, endomorph, or mesomorph—or one's Ayurvedic body type.

We eat clean to support a healthy lifestyle—a clear mind and body makes us less susceptible to emotional swings. If food is fuel, we need to make sure that we are putting in the cleanest, top-grade fuel to run the machine that is our body and mind. We also want to eat foods that will support our serotonin and hormone levels, support our cognitive functions, balance our insulin levels, and enhance our digestion. There is a strong connection to the gut (your gastrointestinal tract) and the brain, a connection referred to as gut-brain axis (GBA). This links to the central nervous system (brain, spinal cord, and gut), and the microorganisms living in your gut play a crucial role in the GBA by producing and expressing neurotransmitters that can affect appetite, mood, or sleep habits; reduce inflammation in your body; and affect cognitive function and your response to stress.

Constipation, gas, bloating, and water retention do nothing for our good mood and contribute to generally feeling bad. Eating foods that work for our unique and individual bodies are key, and developing "lean consciousness" is paramount.

In *YogaLean*, I also illuminate how, through the practice of yoga, we learn to gain a sense of our bodies. By living in "lean consciousness," we learn how to listen to the needs of our bodies so that we make the right choices and stay in optimal health. We then maintain both our physical and mental health through knowledge, practice, belief, and intention.

Focusing on clean eating can truly make a difference in healing trauma, anxiety, and depression. If our gut is unhealthy, then it will not adequately function, not only in producing serotonin, but general nourishment of the mind and body. In addition to keeping our gut happy and healthy, there are certain foods that are beneficial for depression. When developing a healthier relationship with the food you consume, your body begins to function on a more enriched level. For trauma, if your body is absorbing the natural (and diverse) nutrients it needs, then your mind will also be nourished. Clean eating will help you with this.

New research confirms that our mental health declines when we practice poor dietary choices; we can literally become debilitated. More and more, science shows that a diet filled with junk food can lead to poor mental health—such as chronic depression, anxiety, or other forms of psychological distress—making the case that our mood truly depends on food. A diet high in refined sugar contributes to mental struggle and lack of acute concentration. Processed junk food is not only detrimental to the gut due to lack of nutrients, it is often packed with pesticides, chemicals, and addictive additives that can spike inflammation and insulin levels and ultimately weaken organs and bones, not to mention the cognitive dysfunction that comes from refined carbohydrates, gluten, and high blood sugar.

One of the reasons the food you eat determines your mood is because having too much or too little sugar in your blood can be stressful for your brain. From an evolutionary point of view, both are perceived as a threat to your survival. A steep rise in blood sugar gives you a temporary good feeling, which is also known as a sugar high. However, persistent high blood sugar can be dangerous and lead to complications mentally and physically. A slump in blood sugar is what makes you feel lethargic and jumpstarts your adrenals that secrete fight-or-flight hormones. This alone speeds up your breathing, heart, and anxiety.

This is usually when you reach for one or all of the following: chocolate, coffee, a salty carb snack, alcohol, drugs, or cigarettes. It's got very little to do with self-control. The good news is that you can prevent these effects and take better care of your brain by making healthier choices.

Science has linked sugar intake, anxiety, and depression before, however we now know mood disorders often come first. Depressed, anxious, and traumatized people tend to eat more sugar as a result of their mental health issues. Sugar hurts our mental health, and many people struggle with giving it up. Sugar is highly addictive and very hard to give up as people often rely on the daily boosts of feel-good hormones in the brain that come from candy, soda, cookies, and bread.

Food is fuel, and fuel is medicine and can remedy both our moods and chronic ailments that we struggle with. A lot of diseases can be lessened with a cleaner diet. The same goes for depression, anxiety, and PTSD. The related symptoms can all be mitigated with a clean eating program. While at first it may seem difficult to create a new eating regimen, take it one step at a time so that it isn't an overwhelming task. Try not to make it a cumbersome undertaking. Rather, allow it to become one small step in your healing, like mentioned before. Try adding in at first instead of subtracting—for example, "adding in" more flaxseed oil, adding in more leafy greens and orange vegetables.

The following is a list of foods that are good for the overall improvement and maintenance of the mind and body. In YogaFit's level two training, we talk about the concept of "face and replace." We may need to face the facts that our diets are not supporting our healing and then replace food and habits that don't serve us. We replace processed junk for real foods like vegetables, fruits, grass-fed meats, whole grains, healthy fat sources (avocados, nuts, and seeds), and healthier oils such as avocado and olive oil. It also means steering clear of the Standard American Diet (aptly named SAD), which consists of fried foods, factory-farmed and processed meat, fast food, refined grains, pizza, and high-sugar foods and drinks. A good rule of thumb is to eat a variety of colorful fruits and vegetables, which will ensure you're absorbing a diverse range of nutrients that benefit you differently.

Healthy Digestion

Your digestive tract plays a vital role in your physical and mental health and is responsible for absorbing nutrients and eliminating waste. These nutrients enrich your microbiome, which helps your body develop good bacteria to ward off diseases and enhance production of serotonin. If you incorporate foods rich in fiber or probiotics, your digestive tract will function with more ease.

- **Probiotic foods**—dark chocolate, asparagus, garlic, onions, and jicama support gut bacteria.
- **Fermented foods**—yogurt, tempeh, kimchi, kombucha, and sauerkraut are packed-full of probiotics.
- **Apples**—pectin found in apples helps increase bowel movement through your digestive tract. It may also decrease inflammation in your colon.
- **Fennel**—fiber content and an antispasmodic agent can improve digestion by limiting some negative gastrointestinal symptoms.
- **Kefir**—the unique ingredient, "grains" made from yeast and bacteria, appear to improve digestion and decrease inflammation in your gut.
- **Chia Seeds**—fiber content of chia seeds can assist digestion by promoting the growth of probiotics in your gut and keeping you regular.
- **Papaya**—containing papain, which is a strong digestive enzyme that contributes to the healthy digestion of proteins. It may also relieve IBS symptoms.
- **Whole Grains**—Due to their high fiber content, whole grains can support healthy digestion by adding bulk to your stool, reducing constipation, and feeding your healthy gut bacteria.
- **Beets**—nutrients in beets are a strong component to healthy gut

production and movement.

- **Miso**—probiotic content found in miso makes it helpful for reducing digestive issues and overcoming intestinal illness like diarrhea.
- **Bone Broth**—Bone broth is made by simmering the bones and connective tissues of animals. The gelatin found in bone broth can help improve digestion and protect your intestinal wall. It may be useful in improving leaky gut and other inflammatory bowel diseases.
- **Peppermint**—peppermint may ease symptoms of IBS, including bloating, stomach discomfort, and bowel-movement issues due to the oils in peppermint that are seen to have a relaxing effect on the muscles in the digestive tract.

Serotonin and Mood Boosters

Serotonin helps regulate mood, social behavior, appetite, digestion, sleep, memory, and sex drive. The majority of serotonin is produced in our gastrointestinal tract, therefore it's important to feed our bodies with foods that support a healthy gastrointestinal tract.

- **Avocado**—in addition to healthy fats, avocado has Vitamin B6, which helps the body make serotonin and several other neurotransmitters. Avocados are a source of healthy monounsaturated fats that the body can use for energy, and vitamin B, which naturally increases energy levels.
- **Almonds**—in addition to being rich in omega-threes, almonds are also a great source of magnesium. Magnesium is a great way to calm your nervous system. These hearty nuts also contain vitamin E, which is helpful for the immune system.
- **Asparagus**—high in folate, a mood-boosting nutrient, and due to its high levels of vitamin B, you will also feel a surge of good energy when eating asparagus. It supports healthy energy levels by turning carbs into glucose. The low glycemic index of asparagus also means that its energy release is gradual and long-lasting.
- **Blueberries**—in addition to their high antioxidant content, blueberries are also high in vitamin C, which has been shown to help provide relief from anxiety.

- **Garbanzo Beans and Hummus**—help release serotonin and are high in fiber, which is good for gut balance.
- **Saffron**—known in traditional Chinese medicine as *fan hong hua*, this herb is often prescribed for depression. Saffron is said to lift the spirits and calm the nerves. The safranal, an essential oil in the plant, is responsible for the relief for depression. I take it twice per day.
- **Raw Cashews**—jam-packed with minerals and vitamins, high-protein cashews can be a boost of good energy and vitality.

Calming Foods

There are certain foods that calm your nervous system. I find I naturally crave these foods, especially at night. Please note that they are all healthy and relaxing to the system. These are my favorites:

- **Turkey**—contains tryptophan, an amino acid that your body needs to produce serotonin.
- **Starchy foods**—sweet potatoes, yams, plantains, brown rice, quinoa, beans, and lentils are high-fiber slow carbs.
- **Walnuts and flaxseeds**—Foods rich in omega-threes (including nuts, seeds, and fish like sardines and salmon) lower inflammation and have been shown to reduce anxiety scores.
- **Herbal Tea**—L-theanine in tea is a stress-relieving compound that binds to GABA receptors, which help the brain calm down. Teas like chamomile, rooibos, peppermint, and more are wonderful afternoon options when you're feeling erratic.
- **Yogurt**—Researchers from Ireland's University College Cork published a study that links a specific kind of bacteria, called *Lactobacillus rhamnosus* JB-1, to lower levels of stress and anxiety.
- **Bananas**—potassium, an electrolyte that helps the body stay hydrated, is found in bananas. Bananas also contain magnesium, vitamin B6, and other nutrients that help boost production of digestion-enhancing mucous, as well as promote feelings of happiness and calm inside the body. They also aid in the production of serotonin and melatonin, hormones that regulate mood and sleeping patterns.

Cognitive Enhancers

Food can greatly affect our brain's performance, and so can stress and trauma. If you are working from all angles to enhance your brain function, including your dietary choices, then your mental abilities will become stronger. Foods with omega-three fatty acids, B vitamins, and antioxidants are wonderful components, and with those, your heart and blood vessels will also reap the benefits.

- **Leafy Greens**—Leafy greens such as kale, spinach, and collards are rich in brain-healthy nutrients like vitamin K, lutein, folate, and beta carotene. They also play a strong role in healthy digestion by adding fiber and magnesium to your diet.
- **Fatty fish**—Fatty fish are abundant sources of omega-three fatty acids.
- **Berries**—Flavonoids, the natural plant pigments that give berries their brilliant hues, also help improve memory, research shows. They are also jam-packed with vitamin C, which helps cope with cortisol, a hormone that is released during times of stress.
- **Walnuts**—Nuts are excellent sources of protein and healthy fats, and this type of nut in particular might also improve memory.
- **Dark chocolate**—the antioxidants, protein, and fiber in dark chocolate support a positive mood and healthy cognition. Eat in moderation.
- **Fruits**—Apples, bananas, and oranges are packed with fiber and vitamin C.

Energizing Foods

Each of the foods on this list either naturally has caffeine or is high in energizing nutrients like fiber and B12, although there's no way we can really measure if they're "better" than coffee.

- **Caffeine**—in moderation, caffeine will give you a nice boost of energy, but too much of it will give your body a quick spike and then a slump that is hard to recover from, which can cause anxiety.
- **Oatmeal**—the complex carbohydrates in oatmeal will give you slow-burning fuel to keep you energized well into the late morning. It also helps with the production of serotonin.

- **Sesame seeds**—rich in magnesium, a nutrient which helps convert sugar into energy. Sesame seeds also have fiber and healthy fats that help stabilize blood sugar levels.
- **Cinnamon**—a whiff of cinnamon reduces fatigue.
- **Water**—drink a lot of water as it will ward of symptoms of dehydration and will create a healthy flow for your internal organs to function.
- **Dates**—the naturally high sugar content, along with fiber in dates, will give you a natural jolt of energy while also filling you with vitamins.
- **Beans**—beans are rich in complex carbohydrates, fiber, and protein, which promotes a slow, steady rise and fall in blood glucose levels, helping to stabilize energy levels.
- **Watermelon**—filled with vitamin B, magnesium, and potassium, it has naturally energy-boosting properties.
- **Broccoli**—packed with fibers, vitamin A, C, and E, and with antioxidants and chromium, a mineral that helps regulate blood sugar.
- Sardines—a huge source of omega-threes, protein, and vitamin B12, a nutrient essential to converting food into energy
- **Cardamom**—increases circulation and improves energy.
- **Eggs**—rich in protein and B vitamins including B1, B2, B6, and B12, which are essential for energy production. Eggs also contain lecithin and choline needed for proper methylation and nervous-system function. Choline is a nutrient that forms a key part of the abundant neurotransmitter acetylcholine, used all the time for motor and memory functions in the nervous system.
- **Cashews**—rich in magnesium, which works to convert sugar to energy via glycolysis while protein helps keep you full. fiber in dates,

Immune system boosters

A healthy body helps keep you vigilant, full of energy, and able to get you on your feet and do the things you love. When your body is sick and inactive, it ultimately affects brain function, which may lead to feelings of depression.

- **Citrus fruits**—grapefruit, oranges, tangerines, lemons, limes, clementines, etc. Vitamin C is thought to increase the production of white blood cells, which are crucial to the immune system's efforts in fighting off infectious diseases

- **Red bell peppers**—filled with vitamin C and beta carotene. Both not only help your immune system, they promote healthy eyes and skin, too.
- **Garlic**—garlic's immune-boosting properties seem to come from a heavy concentration of sulfur-containing compounds, such as allicin.
- **Ginger**—ginger is a wonder food that helps to decrease inflammation, nausea, chronic pain, and cholesterol.
- **Spinach**—spinach is rich in vitamin C. It's also packed with numerous antioxidants and beta carotene, which may increase the infection-fighting ability of our immune systems.
- **Tea**—both green and black teas are packed with flavonoids, a type of antioxidant.
- **Kiwis**—enriched with folate, potassium, vitamin K, and vitamin C.
- **Sunflower seeds**—sunflower seeds are full of nutrients, including magnesium, phosphorous, and vitamin B6. They're also incredibly high in vitamin E, a powerful antioxidant.
- **Shellfish**—crabs, clams, mussels, and oysters are packed with zinc. Zinc doesn't get as much attention as many other vitamins and minerals, but our bodies need it so that our immune cells can function as intended.

Anti-Inflammation Diet—or What NOT To Eat

On top of adding clean foods into your diet, it's important to eliminate those foods that are bad for you and your internal workings. These include:

- Gluten (it creates brain fog)
- Refined carbohydrates, such as white bread and pastries
- Soda and other sugar-sweetened beverages
- Red meat (burgers, steaks) and processed meat (hot dogs, sausage)
- Margarine, shortening, and lard
- Sugar
- Junk food or fast food
- Excess alcohol or caffeine
- Fried or breaded foods
- Dairy

Here are some additional tips from *Clean Eating* author Lisa Davis:

1. Before you go out and buy the foods in [the deli] section, have a plan. For example,"I will get some turkey and make sure I have whatever I need to go along with it to make sure it gets eaten." If you love whole grain bread and a little mayo, be sure to get that too.

2. Be aware of what is perishable and what doesn't need to be eaten right away. For example,"I will get some almonds that I can easily access, and I will be sure to eat the fresh blueberries today or tomorrow. I will also buy frozen berries that I can use at a later time for smoothies."

3. Look at the foods in [the produce] section and google recipes. For example. "Recipe with asparagus, garlic, and onions."There are so many great recipes that pop up.

4. Keep SAD foods out of the house.

5. If you are not up to cooking every day, buy some canned, frozen, or pre-made meals. Just be sure to check the ingredients to see if they are made with real foods.

6. Do the best you can. Some days, self-care might be tougher than others, and if you are not up for shopping and only have something to eat that isn't the best, it's okay. Do the best you can.

7. Look into meal delivery services. There are a lot of good ones out there where either the meal is fully prepped, or they give you the exact amounts of what you need to make the recipe.

8. Always remember to eat whole foods as much as possible.

9. Also remember to get your complex carbs from veggies, fruits, and whole grains (if you tolerate grains). Be sure to eat healthy protein sources. If you do eat meat, look for grass-fed. Also very important to stay hydrated. Hydration is critical for mental awareness and overall health. The rule of thumb is eight to ten eight-ounce glasses of water per day.

10. If you are vegan or vegetarian you will need to be aware of healthy eating as well. For example potato chips and French fries consumed to excess are just not healthy—neither is gluten-rich pasta. Most meat and poultry sources are now factory-farmed and just not clean.

These animals die in a traumatic way, and that energy is passed along when you consume their flesh. Consider eating a more plant-based diet, but put the cookies down.

Knowing what to eat and the why is only part of the puzzle. The rest is figuring out how to make it work for you. Clean eating will go a long way in your healing, I promise you. Try it for a month and see how you feel as the toxins leave your body. Your mind and emotions will thank you, and so will the vessel that is carrying your spirit around—your beautiful and amazing body.

Survivor story: Sheilah

In 2014, I was diagnosed with stage four throat cancer. I was practicing Ayurveda during my intensive rounds of radiation and chemo. When my cancer returned stage four in 2015, I had to have a radical neck dissection and I continued to practice Ayurveda wellness.

In 2016, while teaching a fitness class, I had a stroke! I found my way to the mat while in hospital, and that's when I asked the universe, "What do you need from me?" The answer was to slow down. That is when I made a commitment to start healing myself. I was so numb and dealing with my own struggles from being numb to everything. PTSD was real for me. I was living in a heightened mind that was forever waiting for the next shoe to drop while dealing with having a brain that didn't work like it once did. I had to learn to forgive myself for my brain injury and that I am now a ten-second thinker in a one-second world.

I went to yoga at a fellow YogaFit instructor's studio and was gifted the ability to heal. I was so grateful for the opportunity that I became a YogaFit instructor. I completed my 500 hours in May of 2019.

I specialized in Warriors. My life was changed. I signed up for the Warriors intensive 2018, and my own healing began. I also completed the 100-Hour Ayurveda and added that into my daily life as well as informed my students of the benefits of healing from the bottom up and from the inside out.

I opened my own studio, and I now run five ten-week Warrior sessions consecutively. One session is only for medical clinicians to ensure they are not with any patients. I have four psychotherapists, two paramedics on medical leave, and two police officers on medical leave.

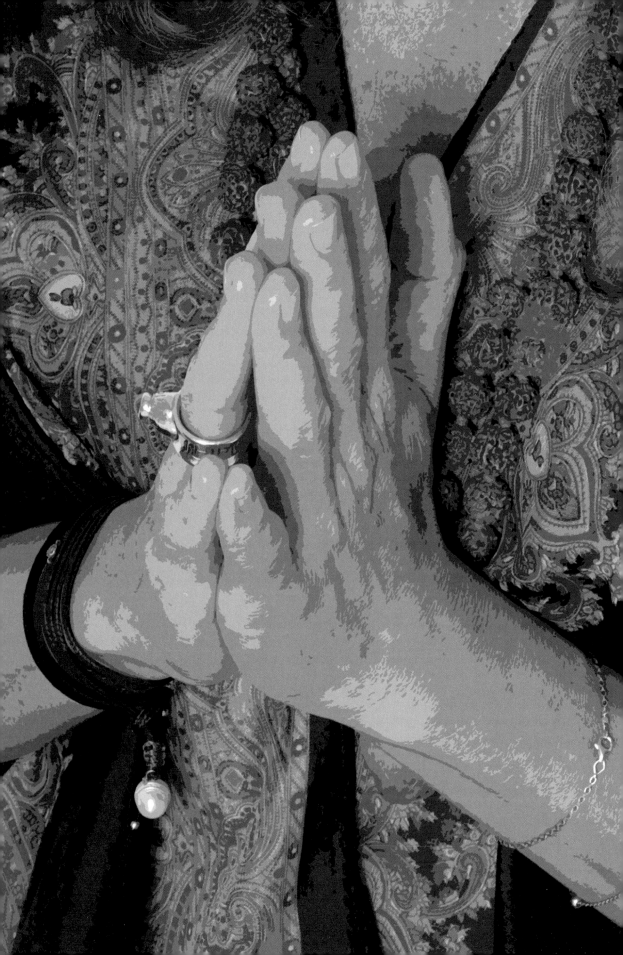

CHAPTER 10

Living Your Best Life: Coping with Trauma and Mitigating Your Symptoms

*"It is better to do your own dharma
[calling] even imperfectly, than
someone else's dharma perfectly."*
—Bhagavad Gita 3:35

*"Those who see through the eye of knowledge the
difference between the field and the knower of the field,
and thus know the means to the living entity's liberation
from material nature attain the Supreme themselves."*
—Bhagavad Gita 13:5

While we may never heal completely from trauma, but we can certainly learn to mitigate and cope with the daily symptoms and feelings. Or as they say in the Twelve-Step Program—"One day at a time."

As we have mentioned—awareness is the key component to managing the day-to-day shifts and storms. My own approach to living with trauma, depression, and emotional dysregulation is simple yet complex. It involves a constant vigilance and being the witness to the body, mind, and emotions. I use intention plus action to get results, and I use the tools in this book daily.

This is where my yoga practice has become crucial. We now know yoga allows us to be the witness to the body, mind, and emotions, and make better choices that contribute to:

- Healthier lifestyle
- Positive mood
- Better relationships
- Improved quality of life
- Balanced living

From the place of being the witness, we can then seek the appropriate treatment with clarity. If we don't learn to act from a "wise mind," as stated in Dialectical Behavior Therapy (DBT), we can easily end up blowing up the bridge while standing on it. While talk therapy has its place, I personally believe in the practical learning skills like the ones taught in Cognitive Behavioral Therapy (CBT) and DBT. Both are based on mindfulness. I have found in particular that DBT skills are helpful to deal with the emotional trauma and ensuing dysregulation that occurred for me from my childhood trauma.

Preparing for Triggers

There are times when you are going to be more susceptible to triggers. Taking care of your body with proper sleep, hygiene, adequate nutrition and exercise, and yoga meditation are key.

You can be more easily triggered when you are:

- Tired
- Stressed
- Overworked physically and mentally
- Lacking enough physical movement
- Exposed to extreme temperatures— too hot, too cold
- Under the effects of excess caffeine or alcohol

If you learn to balance your lifestyle and center your wellness on healing, you may become less susceptible to your triggers. Ladies, when we have PMS, we are much more likely to get triggered. I keep a journal of my cycle and take extra precautions during the ten days leading up to my period. There are a variety of supplements that you can take as well as cyclical pharmaceuticals. PMS has always thrown me into a state of almost extreme reactions, triggers, and enhanced negative emotions. Be the witness to your moods and your need for extra rest and a calm environment during this time of the month.

I also keep a general mood journal daily, which helps me track the good days and the bad days and see what I did on those days to contribute to a more positive mood.

Mindfulness Therapy

DBT integrates mindfulness practice and formal coping skills training, which originally assisted those who met the criteria for Borderline Personality Disorder, but are now used by anyone who struggles with mood regulation. Dysregulated emotions are most often created by trauma, and DBT sessions help clients remove the barriers that get in the way of their goals in order to build a life worth living. DBT skills training helps clients enhance their ability to regulate emotions, be mindful of the present moment, tolerate distress, and maintain effective relationships. DBT individual and skills training sessions often target and reduce:

- Mood swings, up-and-down emotions, and problems with anger
- Impulsive, avoidance, and self-harming behavior
- Interpersonal stress, loneliness, and fears of abandonment
- Sense of emptiness, inadequacy, and not knowing where you fit in
- Difficulties thinking clearly and feeling disconnected
- All-or-nothing thinking and difficulties with change
- Family and relationship conflict

CBT is a form of psychological treatment that has been demonstrated to be effective for a range of problems including depression, anxiety disorders, alcohol and drug use, marital issues, eating disorders, and severe mental illness.

People suffering from psychological problems can learn better ways of coping with them, thereby relieving their symptoms and becoming more effective in their lives. One skill practiced in DBT is proactively seeking out positive moments and experiences and building them into our everyday lives in order build happy feelings. One way to do this is scheduling an activity that will bring you joy; whether that is something as simple as going for ice cream or something more elaborate like a whale-watching trip. Another is to recognize things in your day that make you feel positive emotions—the cool breeze, hearing your favorite song on the radio, or conversing with someone you love.

Take note of the body sensations that are elicited when you experience these things. Also, the mental and emotional response that takes you away from the trauma and brings you into those moments of happiness. It is very helpful to keep a mood journal daily to see what you did on those days to contribute to a more positive mood.

While it is difficult to do this when you are depressed or anxious, being aware of these moments can help you alleviate difficult feelings and develop a more balanced view of the present. Engaging in and identifying enjoyable activities helps retool your thinking to understand that, when things are difficult, there are still other elements that bring joy to your life. And despite your trauma, it is OK to enjoy life now. Being present in the now will help you move forward.

Flow State

The flow state, also known as being in "the zone," was coined by Mihály Csíkszentmihályi in 1975. The concept has been widely cited in positive psychology.

One of the best practices you can engage in to create a bank of positive emotions and find joy in your daily life is to find activities that bring you pure joy and presence, putting you in the "flow state." A flow state is where you are completely immersed in an activity and completely in the present moment of now. When you are engaged in something you love—yoga, dancing, art, playing a musical instrument—you lose track of all time. You become completely focused in an activity and only that activity.

Flow is one of the most enjoyable states of being. It allows us to be present and helps us become more joyous, creative, and productive. For those afflicted with trauma symptoms, it is especially important because your mind lets go of everything except what you are doing: enjoying the present moment. Flow helps us cope with life because focus is associated with better emotion regulation—a crucial skill when coping with negative emotions and memories. When you flow, you tune out distractions, teaching you to move on, to function more effectively and create a strong new network of neural pathways. Flow is the opposite of stagnation. Flow is great for stress management because you feel more competent and take more challenges. Flow helps us be present, set goals, work towards goals, and enjoy your progress and your process. It is such a focused state that your memories don't enter. Another benefit is your inner critic is silenced during this flow state.

The brain, in flow, is more relaxed. Brain waves shift from the beta waves of concentration to the alpha waves associated with rest and relaxation and the theta waves that occur during meditation. Flow enhances learning because it releases dopamine, giving us a sense of excitement. It also helps us notice patterns in the environment by heightening our attention and decreasing distractions. Once those patterns get stored in our memory during the recovery phase after flow, we're able to recognize them in new contexts.

Exercise and Move Your Body

Committing each morning to living your best life takes work, discipline, and an action plan. Personally I find that starting my morning with exercise sets the tone for a great day. I ask my body what it needs in that day— cardio? Weight training? Yoga? Pilates? A brisk walk? A hike? Or maybe just dancing. The endorphins released during movement boost your mood for up to twelve hours, and regular exercise helps ease depression and anxiety while enhancing a sense of well-being. According to the Anxiety and Depression Association of America (ADAA), "psychologists studying how exercise relieves anxiety and depression suggest that a ten-minute walk may be just as good as a forty-five-minute workout." While the relief is brief, over time it can help with an enhanced, prolonged sense of well-being. In one study, researchers found that those who got regular vigorous exercise were twenty-five percent less likely to develop depression or an anxiety disorder over the next five years.

Among the many psychological and emotional benefits, exercise helps with personal power (think of a weight lifter), which builds confidence and encourages social interaction when practiced in a group setting. Creating exercise goals, even small ones, boosts self-confidence and allows you to practice healthy coping skills and makes you want to avoid unhealthy behaviors like drinking, binge eating, and drug use.

Stress and anxiety are simply a part of being human, and anxiety disorders impact forty million adults. Exercise far extends beyond relieving stress, it helps balance your mind and improve anxiety and other disorders related to it. But for those dealing with trauma, PTSD, depression, and anxiety, it's going to be a lot of trial and error. For trauma-sensitive individuals, there are unique exercise concerns to consider.

Taking classes in a gym with heavy weights banging in the next room may be triggering, or going to a class where the instructor makes hands-on adjustments may cause discomfort. I am always sensitive while teaching and notify students that I will be making hands-on adjustments and offer them the opportunity to refuse; pulling on someone's legs in *savasana* (final resting pose) may cause fright and painful memories and destroy the relaxation benefits that we just worked to create. Outdoor exercising near traffic or loud construction may be a trigger for war veterans. Music played too loudly in an exercise class can be too stimulating for those with sensitive nervous symptoms.

How do you know which exercise is best for you? For me the simple answer has always been "try everything and stick with what you love, but continue to try new things." Yes, I love yoga, but I also love weight lifting, cardio (sometimes), Pilates, snowshoeing, hiking, dancing, electric muscle stimulation (EMS), walking, and cycling. When you are depressed, it's often hard to get moving, but this is where finding that one movement that you love so much makes all the difference. I am fortunate because I love exercise; many who do not can learn to love it with enough time, patience, and practice. Starting and sticking with an exercise routine or regular physical activity can be a challenge.

These steps from the Mayo Clinic can help:

- **Identify what you enjoy doing.** Figure out what type of physical activities you're most likely to do and think about when and how you'd be most likely to follow through. For instance, would you be more likely to do some gardening in the evening, start your day with a jog, or go for a bike ride or play basketball with your children after school?

Do what you enjoy to help you stick with it.

- **Get your mental health professional's support.** Talk to your doctor or mental health professional for guidance and support. Discuss an exercise program or physical activity routine and how it fits into your overall treatment plan.

- **Set reasonable goals.** Your mission doesn't have to be walking for an hour five days a week. Think realistically about what you may be able to do and begin gradually. Tailor your plan to your own needs and abilities rather than setting unrealistic guidelines that you're unlikely to meet.

- **Don't think of exercise or physical activity as a chore.** If exercise is just another "should" in your life that you don't think you're living up to, you'll associate it with failure. Rather, look at your exercise or physical activity schedule the same way you look at your therapy sessions or medication—as one of the tools to help you get better.

- **Analyze your barriers.** Figure out what's stopping you from being physically active or exercising. If you feel self-conscious, for instance, you may want to exercise at home. If you stick to goals better with a partner, find a friend to work out with or who enjoys the same physical activities that you do. If you don't have money to spend on exercise gear, do something that's cost-free, such as regular walking. If you think about what's stopping you from being physically active or exercising, you can probably find an alternative solution.

- **Prepare for setbacks and obstacles.** Give yourself credit for every step in the right direction, no matter how small. If you skip exercise one day, that doesn't mean you can't maintain an exercise routine and might as well quit. Just try again the next day. Stick with it.

Dancing

Some days I just put on rap music in the morning and dance for twenty minutes. Dancing is embraced by almost every culture on earth and inherently brings joy. Not only does it spark the endorphins like traditional exercise, it encourages a playful social aspect as well. For some, it triggers an emotional release, whether through laughter, a smile so big it hurts, or tears.

It's cathartic—a letting-go of emotions.

And like other exercise, it boosts the heart rate, reduces stress, and makes you sweat. I love dancing and while I recognize that when depressed no one wants to dance, it may be just the time that you need to dance. Try it for five minutes even when you don't want to. Dancing is truly transformational.

Clear the Clutter

Keeping your life as clean as possible also creates less added stress. You can start with any physical clutter around you; perhaps there are possessions that are triggers from the past. As stated in the Yamas and Niyamas— Cleanliness is paramount and part of your yoga practice.

Make a fearless and ruthless plan that involves clearing anything from your life that is not serving you at this time in your life: this can be possessions or even people.

In rehabs, they say "clean head, clean bed." It's a fact that a clean space, clean living, and clean actions make a person feel better. Just watch an episode of *Hoarders* and you can see firsthand how damaging excess can be.

We learned how clean eating helps avoid and manage stress, anxiety, and depression. We also now have Ayurvedic hacks to practice daily to improve mood and functionality. The bottom line is you must constantly strive to clean up your life on many levels

Giving Back—Service Work

Making a difference matters! Giving back and having a higher purpose goes a long way in leading a meaningful, purposeful life. Helping others gets you out of your own thoughts, pain, depression, and darkness. There are many things you can do on a daily, weekly, and monthly basis to help your community. I urge you to read this list and take the personal challenge to give back on a regular basis. It will help you focus on something other than your own pain. Not only will others benefit, but doing good for others is Karma Yoga, and you will reap the benefits tenfold.

Daily

Volunteer at your local animal shelter or ASPCA to walk orphan dogs.

Volunteer with Meals on Wheels to deliver food to the elderly and infirm.

Weekly

Donate any already-read magazine or books to senior centers or retirement homes.

Monthly

Donate old towels, sheets, and blankets to your local animal shelter or pet rescue organization. Donate pet toys and food too.

Teach a free yoga class to a group of at-risk teens.

Donate body care products to the Visiting Nurse.

Annually

Donate clothes unworn for six months to organizations like men's rehabs or homeless shelters.

Always spay and neuter your pets—save lives and stop overpopulation.

Donate eyeglasses to an organization in need.

Join and offer your time at a twelve-step meeting. Twelve-step meetings are life-changing and will help you interact with people who are trying to heal and be better.

Journaling

Personal journals are an incredibly powerful yet simple means of processing events and circumstances in your life, healing emotional wounds, and moving forward with passion and intention. Your return to health and wellbeing often involves being willing to feel in order to heal. The blank page is a safe, objective audience for fielding memories, thoughts, and emotions—rational or irrational. It holds your hand as you dive into exploring the subconscious and does not pass judgment.

Journaling helps you set goals and also to come to terms with suppressed memories, confusing or traumatic events. Like meditation practices, there are many ways to use a journal, and I encourage you to try as many as possible to discover which are most effective for you. Set a timer for ten to fifteen minutes and write whatever comes to mind, that means positive, negative, and otherwise. A journal allows your emotions, thoughts, and energy to flow onto the page, unchecked by judgments or expectations. Journaling gives you the opportunity to clear the mind of the rigors that cloud your well-being, even if those thoughts look scattered on the page. "Letting go" of those thoughts through journaling will instill a sense of release that overcomes you.

Recording inspiration: Write down quotes, poems, advice, and "aha" moments that come your way. This creative act is healing and will give legs to your intentions.

Prayers: Writing down your prayers is an act of surrender, the fifth niyama, and ultimate relinquishing of control.

Positive Affirmations: Writing your positive affirmations reinforces what yoga calls your sankalpa, or positive resolve. Also, it allows you to go back and reflect on your personal growth and success.

Diagnostic Testing

To really understand your baselines for trauma and associated symptoms, I believe that getting baseline tests are crucial. Blood tests every six months will give you your hormone levels, indicate any vitamin deficiencies and functions that need addressing. If your levels are off, it can throw off your mood, energy level, and even your thought processes.

Electroencephalograms, SPECT scans, and neurofeedback sessions, while expensive, are great diagnostic tools for getting baselines on your brain. In certain cases, insurance companies may cover it.

Handling Triggers

Thoughts create feelings, feelings create behaviors.

PTSD triggers can occur at anytime, anywhere. They can be stimulated by external factors in your environment or, even worse, your own internal thoughts that create feelings. Certain thoughts, feelings, and situations can bring up PTSD symptoms, such as memories of the traumatic event, anxiety, depression, terror, and fear. A good way for you to cope with this is to increase our awareness of these triggers. You also need to understand the impact of your neural pathway wiring and your own potential addiction to peptides that are released when you think certain thoughts. By understanding what thoughts, feelings, and situations are our own personal or potential triggers, you can gain a lot more control over them.

Through mind-body practices—your yoga, meditation, mindfulness, breathing, exercise, and Ayurveda—you can limit their occurrence and impact. You learn to get out of PTSD states more rapidly with your new tools. You can also make a conscious choice to avoid those triggers. For example if someone was mugged in a dark alley, they will know to avoid dark alleys. The body does not know the difference between a perceived and real threat. In my book, *The YogaFit Athlete*, you used guided imagery to imagine winning a game, race, or making the perfect shot. The darker side of the mind creates tremendous stress for the entire system when you let it create reoccurrences of the cause of your trauma or fears of future trauma. The mind will protect itself at all costs, which can actually cost us everything.

Types of Triggers

There are two types of triggers: external and internal. External covers those occurrences outside of the body, including people, places, and situations. While internal are those things that come from within, like thoughts, memories, pain, and feelings.

External Triggers
- Anniversaries, holidays, birthdays
- Locations and places

- Watching the news may remind you of your traumatic event
- Watching a movie that sparks your traumatic event
- Falls and car accidents
- Smells and sounds
- The end of a relationship
- A specific place
- Seeing the person who caused your trauma

Internal Triggers:

- Memories
- Dreams or nightmares
- Thoughts
- Feelings
- Sensations
- Headaches or Migraines
- Body Aches
- Racing heartbeat
- Shortness of breath
- Feeling out of control
- Pain and Muscle Tension

Seven Steps to Take Control of Your Triggers

Here are a few things you can proactively do to alleviate, control, and—maybe with time—avoid your personal triggers.

1. Know and understand your own emotional and physical triggers.
2. Spot and avoid external stimuli.
3. Identify internal causes
4. Acceptance and non-judgement—Use the YogaFit Essence of breathing and feeling
5. Journal daily
6. Have healthy coping skills
7. Practice neurofeedback and meditation

Support Groups

When dealing with trauma or PTSD, finding your "tribe" can be life-altering. Getting a strong support group of people who can share their life experience with you is priceless. A supportive community shows you that you are not alone in your struggles, nor are you unique in your experience. Community gives you the opportunity to help yourself by helping others and to get comfortable being yourself by revealing your story to those who have experienced perhaps not the same exact story but suffer just the same. I truly believe in the twelve-step model. I find AA meetings to be very inspirational. As a sobriety coach, I highly encourage daily twelve-step meetings. Whether you are going to a twelve-step to stay sober, stay off drugs, stop gambling, rid yourself of a love addiction, cease a shopping or gambling habit, or are even drowning in clutter (Hoarders Anonymous)—there is a twelve-step program for you. I even heard from a vegan friend that there is a "Carnivores Anonymous" meeting in LA for those who are trying (and struggling) with being or staying vegetarian.

I am fortunate to have a strong supportive network of friends that I can be honest and open with. Sometimes we get together for Goddess Gatherings or Vision Board Parties. These are fun, bonding, and allow you to open up in a safe place.

Additional Ways to Get Unstuck:

Writing this book forced me to get stuck and unstuck. A project that has not only consumed a lot of my time but obviously forced me to deal with a lot of my own issues around my own personal life experience and trauma as well. Not to mention my struggles with writer's block and procrastination. I have even gone so far as to cover my TV with a sheet in order to avoid distractions. Unfortunately, my distractions also include a massive travel schedule, work, working out, compulsive organizing (OCD), and a tendency towards "hyper socializing," as one friend put it.

On a darker side, my distractions involve bad reality TV and even worse amazon Prime movies—hence the covered screen. We all have ways that we distract ourselves, some healthier than others. Even with awareness, we can still participate in the behavior.

Here are twenty-two ways (besides yoga) that I use to get motivated when I feel stuck:

1. Mantras on YouTube going constantly in the background at my home—sound waves permeate your walls, your space, and you. Having mantras playing is calming and clears the space, infusing positive energy. I play the *Bhagavad Gita* a few times a week, and mantras almost every day and sometimes even while I sleep.

2. A long walk with my dog or a trip to the dog park to just enjoy dog joy. There is an unbridled joy that animals bring. They exist in the now, don't get distracted by social media, and are very present and alert. The act of caring for a pet that gives unconditional love will bring immense joy (especially if you rescued the animal). I love walking with Bentley and taking him to play as it forces me to be present.

3. A spray bottle with essential oils that I spritz on my face (note: keep your eyes closed when you do this). I use scents a lot; they lift my spirits and refresh me. We offer some amazing sprays and oils through YogaFit. My favorite day spray is either cinnamon and clove or peppermint and eucalyptus. My go-to night-time spray is lavender and patchouli. I also like a lemon fresh for my car and sandalwood for anytime.

4. A quick workout with very heavy weights to change up my energy. Weight lifting literally shifts your hormones—a leg workout can raise your testosterone and growth hormone levels—switching your mood within twenty-five minutes.

5. A headstand. Inversions are known for their mood lifting benefits. They allow you to turn things around and upside down. They spark the nervous system and allow blood flow to the brain, eyes, face, neck, and scalp. To make a headstand more accessible and supportive, try the original Headstander BodyLift Headstand Bench from Evolution Health. See Appendix for coupon code.

6. A guided meditation with a weighted blanket. What a great combo. I love my weighted blanket; it's like getting a big hug. Weighted blankets are proven to reduce anxiety. They ease insomnia and help with

attention deficit disorder and sensory processing disorder. I have one that weighs seventeen pounds and use it a few times a week for meditation and often to sleep. I love my blanket from Magic Weighted Blanket. See Appendix for coupon code. For guided meditation technology that senses your brainwave activity to focus your attention back to your breath, try the Muse headband. Muse technology is being used in hundreds of hospitals and universities worldwide, including Yale, Harvard, MIT, IBM, and NASA. Research has documented other benefits, like increased grey matter density, reduced thinning of the prefrontal cortex, decreasing amygdala activity (associated with stress response), and increased resilience—basically and overall beneficial change of the brain's structure and function. *See Additional Resources for a coupon code.*

7. Turn off and cover the TV. Benefits include weight loss, reduction in mindless eating. This can lead to better relationships and higher self-esteem.

8. Put the phone away at least one day a week. Benefits include less distractions, staying in the present moment, and more sleep—the light from the phone interrupts sleep.

9. Alternating hot and cold showers or cryotherapy. This resets the nervous system and helps reduce inflammation, pain, and anxiety. It also reduces depression and migraines and recharges you.

10. Taking cognitive enhancers like MCT oil. It helps increase my concentration, focus, and productivity. With moderation, stimulants like coffee can make you feel more "up."

11. Listening to Oprah's Super Soul Sundays or podcasts on inspiration and productivity. Inspiration and motivation lead to transformation.

12. A diet heavy in fruits and vegetables. You will feel lighter, clearer, and cleaner. Foods rich in fiber, vitamins, and minerals will make you healthier.

13. The twelve-step serenity prayer. I spontaneously say this to myself often. It's become one of my mantras. "God grant me the serenity to accept the things I cannot change, the courage to change the things I can, and the wisdom to know the difference."

14. Allowing myself some organizing time every day but not too much. I

have a bit of OCD, but it can get out of control, so I have to limit myself. Compulsive organizing actually is a self-soothing mechanism, but at least things stay in order.

15. Making giant post-it notes on my walls with goals, projects and a to-do list so I see it daily. Stay on top of your goals by looking at them.

16. Time with friends. A great way to laugh, smile, and share, this fun activity changes your energy.

17. Red light therapy. It feeds your cells, increases energy, rejuvenates skin tone, and decreases inflammation. You can buy small handheld units online or visit a Korean spa that will have a full infrared room.

18. Keep a notebook with action items, thoughts, ideas, and projects. This helps in keeping you inspired, on track, organized and gives you accountability. Helps with remembering things and charting your progress.

19. Drink half an ounce of water for every pound you weigh. For example: A 140-pound person should drink seventy ounces of water a day. This helps brain function and energy levels, reduces stress, and improves physical performance.

20. Be vigilant with time; don't let anyone steal it. Our time is all we really have. Feel less overwhelmed by saying "no" unless you really want to say yes. Enjoy more time for rest and relaxation, meditation and exercise, and just doing your favorite things.

21. Enjoy a salt lamp. It increases serotonin levels, neutralizes the energy of your space, and purifies the air.

22. Sleep better at night by blocking harmful "junk light" from your life. Junk light suppresses your body's ability to create melatonin, the sleeping- and waking-cycle regulator in your body. "We absorb this light from our smartphone screens, computer monitors, and LEDS and CFL artificial lights that are all over our environments." Products like True Dark glasses can remove or filter this light which can be the cause of eye strain, headaches, short-term memory loss, stress, anxiety, and depression so you can rest better. *See Appendix for coupon code.*

Living your best life requires daily practice. It requires that you show up, be present for yourself, and take action. Remember that only intention plus action creates results. I tell my staff this constantly.

Some days will feel impossible and others will be smooth. Such is the flow of life. Remember that your soul chose your body and your life experiences to grow and transform, and unfortunately, we all grow more through pain than pleasure.

Initially I did not want to write this book. In fact I gave my new publisher seven titles, and this was the one that they chose.

I recognize that I did not want to write it because I knew I would have to share my own trauma story if I was asking others to share theirs.

Despite being a somewhat well-known person, I am also a very private one. I don't let people into my inner headspace, thought processes, or—in particular—my emotional landscape very easily. Writing this book has forced me to be courageous, open, and bold. I hope that, like myself, you will let your trauma rip your heart open and keep that heart open, because an open heart grows and blooms. An open heart also has compassion and sensitivity and understands the suffering of the world. Continue to help heal others and grow your heart.

I also knew I still needed to connect the dots on some of my own trauma and how it has affected and continues to affect my life. I would be lying if I said this was an easy book to write, to get out and to complete. I struggled every step of the way. I'd like to acknowledge the brave souls who chose to share their stories with you through this book. We heal what gets revealed. Thank you for giving me the opportunity to write this book, to share and open up. May this book be as healing for you as it is for me. We all heal in different ways and what is most important is that we recognize our victories towards that goal. Celebrate your progress, be kind and loving to yourself. May you have more sunny days than rainy, and if it is rainy ones—and if it rains—dance in that rain!

As my friend Snatam Kaur says in the chant I play at the end of every yoga class I teach -

"Peace to all, love to all, life to all."

Love, Light, and Namaste

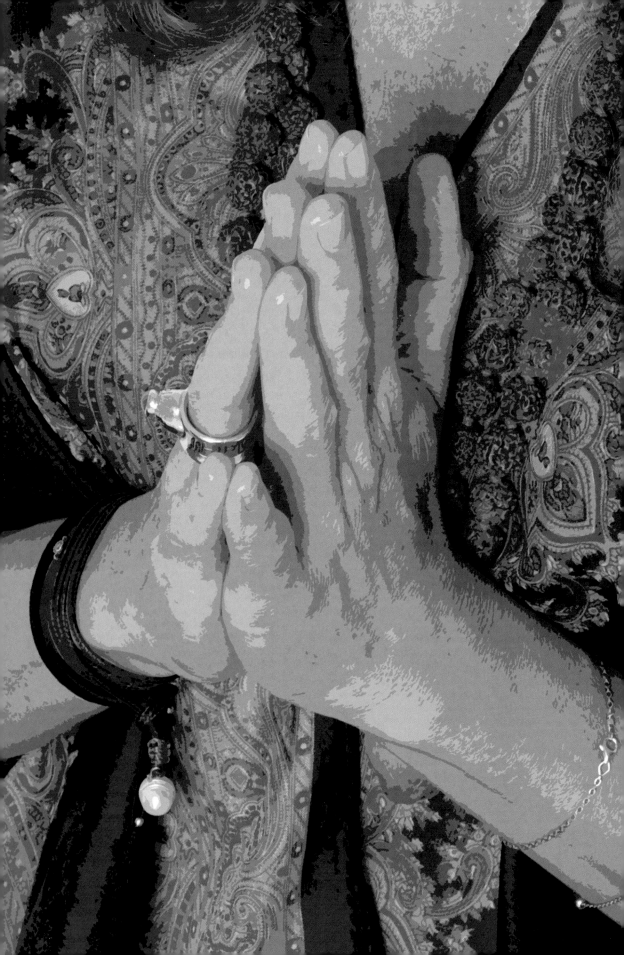

CHAPTER 11

Additional Resources

Anxiety and Depression Association of America. 2018. *Exercise for Stress and Anxiety.* Accessed July 3, 2019. https://adaa.org/living-with-anxiety/managing-anxiety/exercise-stress-and-anxiety.

Desbordes, Gaëlle, Lobsang T. Negi, Thaddeus W. W. Pace, B. Alan Wallace, Charles L. Raison, and Eric L. Schwartz. 2012. "Effects of Mindful-Attention and Compassion Meditation Training on Amygdala Response to Emotional Stimuli in an Ordinary, Non-meditative State." *Frontiers in Human Neuroscience.*

Emerson, David, and Elizabeth Hopper. 2011. *Overcoming Trauma through Yoga: Reclaiming Your Body.* Berkeley, California: North Atlantic Books.

Khalsa, Dharma Singh, and Cameron Stauth. 2001. *Meditation as Medicine: Activate the Power of Your Natural Healing Force.* New York, New York: Simon and Schuster.

Koch, Liz. 2012. *Core Awareness.* Berkeley, California: North Atlantic Books.

Kolk, Bessel A. van der. 2015. *The Body Keeps the Score.* New York, New York: Penguin Books.

Levine, Peter. 2010. *In an Unspoken Voice.* Berkeley, California: North Atlantic Books.

Mayo Clinic. 2017. *Depression and Anxiety: Exercise Eases Symptoms.* September 27. Accessed July 3, 2019. https://adaa.org/living-with-anxiety/managing-anxiety/exercise-stress-and-anxiety.

Scaer, Robert. 2007. *The Body Bears the Burden: Trauma, Dissociation, and Disease.* Philadelphia, Pennsylvania: Haworth Medical Press.

Shaw, Beth. 2016. *The YogaFit Athlete.* New York, New York: Ballantine Books.

—. 2014. *Yoga Lean*. New York, New York: Ballantine Books.

—. 2016. *YogaFit*. Champaign, Illinois: Human Kinetics.

Sounds True. 1999. *Healing Trauma: Restoring the Wisdom of the Body*. Comp. Peter Levine.

Streeter, CC, PL Gerberg, RB Saper, DA Ciraulo, and RP Brown. 2012. "Effects of Yoga on the Autonomic Nervous System, Gamma-Aminobutyric-Acid, and Allostasis in Epilepsy, Depression, and Post-Traumatic Stress Disorder." *Med Hypothesis* 571–9.

Weintraub, Amy. 2012. *Yoga Skills for Therapists*. New York, New York: W. W. Norton.

Attend Twelve-Step Meeting or Other Support Groups

Twelve-step programs are a fellowship of people helping other people with an addiction or a compulsive behavior to obtain abstinence, which means no longer using a mood-altering substance such as drugs or alcohol, or compulsively doing a behavior such as gambling or sex.

Alcoholics Anonymous (AA) was the first twelve-step program established, and many other support groups have branched off from AA using this model. AA is an organization that unites people who have struggled with alcohol dependency, providing strength and faith in one another to overcome addiction. Its mission is to "stay sober and help other alcoholics to achieve sobriety" without judgment or segregation. AA founders Bill Wilson and Dr. Bob Smith developed the twelve steps based on concepts from Carl Jung's theories as influenced by Eastern philosophy, and from spiritual values such as those rooted in the principles of the Oxford Group.

Alcoholics Anonymous and Narcotics Anonymous (NA) are the two largest twelve-step programs available throughout the US. Other programs include:
- Chemical dependency (AA, NA, Pill Addicts Anonymous, Cocaine Anonymous)
- Compulsive gambling (Gamblers Anonymous)

- Eating disorders (Overeaters Anonymous, Food Addicts Anonymous)
- Nicotine addiction (Smokers Anonymous)
- Sexual addiction (Sex and Love Addicts Anonymous, Sex Addicts Anonymous, Sexaholics Anonymous, Sexual Compulsive Anonymous)
- Family and relational issues (Al-Anon, Alateen, Adult Children of Alcoholics, Co-Dependents Anonymous).

Twelve-step programs promote the following fundamental beliefs:
- Addicts require the support of other recovering addicts.
- Reliance on a "power greater than one's self" is fundamental.
- Abstaining from the addictive behavior is the basis of recovery.
- Recovery is a lifelong process.
- Supporting others in recovery is necessary for lasting commitment and stability.
- Accepting the limitations of being human is essential.

The twelve steps, created by AA and first published in 1939, are:
1. We admitted we were powerless over alcohol [addictive substance or behavior]—that our lives had become unmanageable.
2. Came to believe that a Power greater than ourselves could restore us to sanity.
3. Made a decision to turn our will and our lives over to the care of God *as* we understood Him.
4. Made a searching and fearless moral inventory of ourselves.
5. Admitted to God, to ourselves, and to another human being the exact nature of our wrongs.
6. Were entirely ready to have God remove all these defects of character.
7. Humbly asked Him to remove our shortcomings.
8. Made a list of all persons we had harmed, and became willing to make amends to them all.
9. Made direct amends to such people wherever possible, except when to do so would injure them or others.
10. Continued to take personal inventory and, when we were wrong, promptly admitted it.

11. Sought, through prayer and meditation, to improve our conscious contact with God, as we understood Him, praying only for knowledge of His will for us and the power to carry that out.

Having had a spiritual awakening as the result of these steps, we tried to carry this message to alcoholics, and to practice these principles in all our affairs.

I find one of my most significant mantras to be the Serenity Prayer which is recited at the end of every twelve-step meeting:

"God, grant me the serenity to accept the things I cannot change, the courage to change the things I can, and wisdom to know the difference."

This prayer comes to me almost daily. While we cannot change what happened to us in the past, we can change today, and the positive choices we make today lead us to a better tomorrow.

Coupon Codes

COMPANY	WEBSITE	DISCOUNT	CODE
EVOLUTION HEALTH	Evolutionhealth.com	$15 off	yogafit15
LIFECYKEL	lifecykel.com	10% off	YogaFit10
MAGIC WEIGHTED BLANKET	Weightedmagicblanket.com	10% off	YF10
ORGANIC INDIA	organicindiausa.com	20% off	YogaFit20
TRUEDARK	Truedark.com	10% off	YogaFit10
True Hope	Truehope.com	10% off	YogaFit123
UPRIGHT GO POSTURE TRAINER	Uprightpose.com	10% off	YogaFit10
YOGAFIT	Yogafit.com	10% off trainings & conferences	Healing10

Banyan

Lunya $20 off

TrueBrain

Muse 5% off

A warm hug of gratitude to the following special people for their contributions to *Healing Trauma with Yoga:*

Shaye Molendyke for creating the YogaFit Warriors Program and leading the team for trauma healing for first responders at YogaFit Training Systems Worldwide; Kim Gray for editing, researching, and a lot of reading; Felicia Tomasko for instigating Ayurveda at YogaFit and contributing Ayurveda knowledge to this book; Kristin Mabry for her contributions to YogaFit's Level Four and the Healing of Music portion of this book; Lisa Davis for contributing to the Clean Eating chapter; Luciana Pampalone for taking amazing photos; Claudia Micco for reading and feedback. Gabrielle Shaw for family editing and advice; Jenny Baldwin for keeping everything organized at YogaFit; and Danielle Bernabe for being my editor for this book—again!

An extra special thank you to Bentley Shaw for constant canine companionship; the YogaFit Family of master trainers, staff, students, and friends; and my friends who are my chosen family—I truly love and appreciate you.

Thank you to my mother June Shaw for doing the best you could do.

Thank you to my coaches and spirit team.

Finally, I send my appreciation to all of the special souls who came into my life during this process of writing this book and to those who left—thank you, thank you. Thank you for creating the space, God, the universe, and my spirit guides who have had my back and stand beside me even when I haven't supported myself. Thank you for music, prayer, chanting, and the joy of good health.

Peace to all.

Life to all.

Love to all.

Namaste,

Beth